Case Presentations in General Surgery

Other titles published

Case Presentations in Renal Medicine
Case Presentations in Paediatrics
Case Presentations in Cardiology
Case Presentations in Gastrointestinal Disease

Titles in preparation

Case Presentations in Clinical Geriatric Medicine
Case Presentations in Urology

Case Presentations in General Surgery

T. V. Taylor, MD, ChM, FRCS(Eng), FRCS(Ed)
Consultant Surgeon, Manchester Royal Infirmary

C. P. Armstrong, MD, FRCS(Eng), FRCS(Ed)
Senior Registrar, Derriford Hospital, Plymouth

R. N. P. Carroll, FRCS(Eng), FRCS(Ed)
Consultant Urologist, Manchester Royal Infirmary

Butterworths
London Boston Durban Singapore Sydney Toronto Wellington

First published, 1987

© Butterworth & Co. (Publishers) Ltd, 1987

British Library Cataloguing in Publication Data

Taylor, T. Vincent
   Case presentations in general surgery.
   1. Pathology, Surgical——Case studies
   I. Title II. Armstrong, C. P.   III. Carroll, R. N. P.
   617'.07'0926   RD57

   ISBN 0-407-00545-5

Library of Congress Cataloguing in Publication Data

Taylor, T. Vincent.

   Case presentations in general surgery.

   Includes index.
   1. Surgery—Case studies.   2. Surgery—Examinations,
questions, etc.   I. Armstrong, C. P.   II. Carroll, R. N. P.
III. Title.   [DNLM: 1. Surgery—case studies.
2. Surgery—examination question.   WO 18 T246c]
RD34.T35   1986   617   86–32645
ISBN 0-407-00545-5

Phototypesetting by En to En, Tunbridge Wells
Printed and bound in Great Britain by Anchor Brendon Ltd, Tiptree, Essex

Preface

This book is primarily intended for students preparing for professional examinations in surgery. It covers the clinical spectrum of cases predominantly encountered in examinations such as the final MB or final FRCS. The patients described might be considered suitable for major cases or long cases in these examinations, and are used as a basis for the discussion of practical problems encountered in the investigation and management of such cases. The subject matter includes gastroenterological surgery, endocrinology, vascular surgery and urology. A brief history and clinical findings are presented, together with questions relating to investigation and further management. In the discussion following, factors for and against varying forms of management have been compared and contrasted where pertinent.

This text is not comprehensive but may be valuable as an adjunct to a formal work or as an easily read, concise source of revision. We are grateful to Mrs Anita Woodward for typing the text.

T. V. Taylor
C. P. Armstrong
R. N. P. Carroll

Contents

Case Presentations

A 71-year-old man presented with a 3-month history of increasing pain on the left side of the mouth. This was associated with development of an ulcer on the edge of the tongue. Recently he had had difficulty in articulating with concomitant slurring of speech. Occasional small episodes of bleeding were noticed from this ulcer. In his past medical history he had been a heavy smoker, and he drank alcohol in excess.

On examination, he was a thin wasted man. Examination of the mouth revealed an ulcer 2 cm in diameter on the left lateral border of the tongue. This appeared to extend beneath the tongue resulting in a degree of tethering of the tongue itself. The rest of the tongue appeared normal, as did the mucous membranes of the mouth. Examination of the neck revealed enlarged glands in the left anterior triangle which were most prominent just below the jaw. The rest of the examination was unremarkable, apart from the presence of heavy nicotine staining on the fingers.

Investigations

Chest X-ray normal. X-ray of mandible normal. Full blood count and clinical chemistry normal. Serological tests for syphilis were negative.

1

Questions

Discuss the pathology of this condition?
What forms of treatment are available?

Discussion

The most likely diagnosis in this patient with the above history and clinical findings is that of carcinoma of the tongue. Other conditions producing ulcers on the tongue are those of infective glossitis, syphilitic ulcers, aphthous ulcers and lichen planus. Occasionally, benign tumours of the tongue such as adenomas may occur, and salivary gland tumours may be difficult to differentiate from tongue lesions.

Carcinoma of the tongue is almost entirely of the squamous histological type although, rarely, adenocarcinomas can occur. Carcinoma of the tongue accounts for 15% of all malignancies of the head and neck; 80% of cases occurring in men, most being found in patients over 60 years of age. Tumours of the posterior third of the tongue are generally classified as oropharyngeal in origin in contrast to those of the anterior two thirds of the tongue which are classified as true carcinomas of the tongue.

The various predisposing factors associated with the development of carcinoma of the tongue include consumption of spirits, smoking, syphilis, sepsis within the mouth and sharp teeth. It is important to examine the dentition carefully since a sharp tooth may produce a very similar appearance on the tongue to a neoplasm. Several pre-malignant conditions within the oral cavity are currently recognised; the most important of these is leukoplakia. This is characterised by the development of a white plaque on the oral mucosa which cannot be removed easily by rubbing. In this condition pathological changes include widening of the epidermis in association with lymphocyte infiltration into the dermis. Only 4–6% of areas of leukoplakia undergo malignant transformation, nevertheless it is important to examine these areas frequently and to biopsy them.

Erythroplasia is another pre-malignant condition seen on the tongue. This has the appearance of a velvety red, indurated area. Histological examination of biopsy from this area generally reveals carcinoma *in situ* or severe epithelial dysplasia.

The normal clinical appearance of carcinoma of the tongue is that of a chronic, non-healing painless ulcer within the mouth. The presence of pain and difficulty in speaking are generally recognised as advanced symptoms of a rapidly progressing carcinoma.

Carcinoma of the tongue initially spreads via the lymphatics, although blood stream spread also occurs ultimately. Early spread to the submaxillary and the digastric lymph nodes occurs; and, dependent upon the area of the tongue involved, the jugular omohyoid, submandibular and the submental lymph nodes may become involved with secondary tumour deposits.

This patient had definite lymph node involvement within the submandibular lymph glands. Most carcinomas of the tongue occur on the anterolateral side of the tongue, tumours on the dorsum and in the midline being rare. One third of all cases have clinical involvement of nodes on presentation. However, there is a tendency for the tumour to remain in the primary site for many months before spreading to the lymph nodes, and later still to lungs and bone. The absence of palpable lymphadenopathy does not, however, exclude the presence of metastatic disease, since one half of patients without palpable nodes have involvement on microscopic examination.

Carcinoma of the tongue is staged by the tumour, node, metastasis (T.N.M.) classification. 'T' stage is related to the size of the tumour; T1 is less than 2 cm, T2 2–4 cm, T3 greater than 4 cm, T4 greater than 4 cm with deep invasion. Nodal involvement is classified as N0 or N1. Distant bloodborne metastases are classified M1.

Another system of staging which has been used is that where the tumours are graded into stages I, II, III and IV. Stage I are small tumours of less than 2 cm, Stage II tumours of 2–4 cm without lymph node involvement, Stage III tumours with lymph node involvement and Stage IV large tumours with deep invasion with or without distant metastases. The presence of lymph node involvement is approximately related to the size of the primary tumour, thus T1 tumours have 30% positive lymph node involvement, in T2 tumours 50% of lymph nodes are involved and with T3 tumours 70% have involved lymph nodes. Most patients on presentation are in Stages II and III, only 20% being early T1 or Stage I tumours.

The patient described here had a T2 tumour on size alone and the presence of lymph node involvement, without any evidence of distant metastases makes this a T2 N1 lesion. However, fixation of the tongue, with a degree of ankylosis, makes this tumour a T4 lesion. The final staging of this patient, therefore, is Stage III, with a poor prognosis. Initially the diagnosis must be confirmed. The tongue should be biopsied, either under local or general anaesthetic and a wedge taken from the edge of the ulcer. This is carefully examined under the microscope when the diagnosis will almost certainly be that of a squamous cell carcinoma. It is important to exclude syphilis and this can be done by serological testing. The presence of distant metastases should be excluded by means of chest X-ray and bony X-ray if any pain is present.

Once the diagnosis is made, treatment is dependent upon the stage of the tumour. T1 or Stage I tumours can be treated either by partial glossectomy or by radiotherapy. Surgery is much easier with small, anterior tumours and, following such resections, restricted tongue mobility and slurring of speech are minimal. More posteriorly situated larger tumours are associated with a degree of impairment of speech following partial glossectomy. Radiotherapy can be carried out by beam or by implants of radium needles or Radon seeds. T2 tumours may be treated by surgery and occasionally skin grafts in the form of cheek flaps are needed to cover defects. Radiotherapy may also be used in such patients. Following surgery, there is nearly always a degree of speech impairment. Those patients also require ipsilateral neck dissection whereby lymph nodes in the anterior triangle of the neck are removed en bloc. The operation of radical node dissection of the neck is one accompanied with considerable morbidity with complications such as carotid artery bleeding, jugular vein thrombosis, skin flap necrosis and cranial nerve damage being frequently observed. T3 tumours and Stage III disease require radical surgery with associated radiotherapy. Involvement of the mandible may necessitate hemimandibulectomy. Cervical node dissection should be carried out on the ipsilateral side in all patients. This operation has been referred to as a 'Commando' operation.

T4 and Stage IV tumours are beyond surgical help and these patients are best managed by radiotherapy. Chemotherapy has, as yet, little part to play in the management of carcinoma of the tongue although some encouraging results have been reported with the use of agents such as Methotrexate.

The 5-year survival rate of patients with carcinoma of the tongue is overall 40–50%. Stage 1 − 70% 5-year survival; Stage II − 50% 5-year survival; Stage III − 35% 5-year survival and Stage IV − less than 10% 5-year survival. These figures vary from centre to centre, possibly as a result of differences in clinical staging.

The patient described presently had a partial glossectomy, radical lymph node dissection and associated radiotherapy. Happily, the mandible was not found to be involved with tumour and so could be preserved.

Case 2

A 21-year-old female student presented with a 1-year history of dysphagia. Initially intermittent and mild in nature and equally troublesome for liquids and solids, the dysphagia had become more severe over the immediate past 3 months. During the latter period, the patient had been subject to bouts of acute dyspnoea with coughing attacks, particularly when supine. She had also lost half a stone in weight. There was no past medical history of note and no abnormalities present on clinical examination.

Questions

How should this patient be investigated?
What is the likely diagnosis and treatment?

Discussion

This history in a young female is suggestive of achalasia. The initial radiological investigation of this patient should be chest X-ray and barium swallow. Thereafter endoscopy, manometry and 24-hour pH recordings would be helpful possibly together with isotope transit studies. A plain chest X-ray showed a fluid level in the mediastinum and the transverse oesophageal diameter had reached 8 cm. There were signs of consolidation at the lung bases on inspiration. The barium swallow test revealed a markedly dilated mid-oesophagus, with a fluid level smoothly tapering down to a narrow segment over the lower 4-5 cm, thus representing the achalasic segment where there is absence of ganglia in Auerbach's plexus. Endoscopy may show residual fluid or food content in the oesophagus and a degree of oesophagitis; the lower oesophagus usually being quite easily negotiated by the endoscope. Manometry showed a high pressure area in the mid-oesophagus with a relative absence of peristaltic contractions; there was increased pressure in the achalasic segment with failure of relaxation. In this condition ambulatory 24-hour pH studies show an absence of reflux episodes and a constant and usually a neutral oesophageal pH. Antispasmodics such as Octyl nitrate may cause the lower oesophagus to relax.

The patient is treated either by pneumatic dilatation of the lower oesophagus or by surgery. In pneumatic dilatation, an inflatable bag with an outer nylon coat is inflated to a pressure of 300 mmHg inside the achalasic segment and then subsequently deflated. Although the process can be repeated, frequent recurrences are common and the majority of patients have to undergo surgery. Heller's operation performed through an abdominal approach is the treatment of choice. The lower 10 cm of oesophagus are myotomised from the oesophago-gastric junction, proximally. It is important to divide all of the inner circular layer of muscle along the myotomised segment exposing the underlying submucosa. Since a small proportion of patients develop symptoms of gastro-oesophageal reflux following myotomy, some surgeons routinely perform an anti-reflux procedure; however, the author does not subscribe to this view-point as significant reflux occurs in only about 2% of cases. The results of surgery are good, but a small proportion of patients develop recurrence of their achalasia at a later date, and may require a second myotomy, which should then be performed using a transthoracic approach. As there is an increased incidence of carcinoma of the oesophagus in patients with achalasia, which probably persists after surgical treatment, these patients require long-term follow-up.

Case 3

A 43-year-old man presented with a 1-year history of heartburn and regurgitation of food into the mouth. His symptoms were exacerbated by bending and lying down and were associated with flatulence and abdominal distension. On occasions, he was aware of pain radiating posteriorly into the interscapular area. On examination he was found to be moderately overweight, but no abnormal clinical signs were present.

Questions

What is the diagnosis?
How should the patient be investigated?
What methods of treatment are available?

Discussion

The most likely diagnosis is one of gastroesophageal reflux; however, the possibility of peptic ulceration and gallstones should be excluded.

Endoscopic examination of the oesophagus, stomach and duodenum is mandatory. Distal oesophagitis manifests itself by erythematous tongues of inflamed mucosa, erosions and possibly stricture formation. A hiatus hernia may be observed both on introduction and reversed manipulation of the endoscope (J-manoeuvre). Peptic ulceration should be excluded together with malignancies of the lower oesophagus and stomach. A barium swallow and meal are useful in assessing oesophageal motility (tertiary contraction waves may be seen), stricture formation, hiatus hernia and also gastro-oesophageal reflux. Absence of reflux on a barium meal examination does not exclude the diagnosis as, even on provocation by tilting the patient, reflux is not always demonstrated. Indeed, reflux tends to be a variable and intermittent phenomenon. Oesophageal manometry should be performed to identify the site of the problem, and to measure the pressure within the lower oesophageal sphincter. Probably the most valuable adjunct to endoscopy is the measurement of 24-hour ambulatory oesophageal pH. A pH probe is passed to a point 5 cm proximal to the lower oesophageal sphincter and left *in situ,* with the other end strapped to the side of the patient's face for 24-hours during which normal activities are carried out. The recording device, attached to the patient's waist, yields information which may be computerised or played back onto a chart over a period of a few minutes. The number, duration and frequency of reflux episodes (below pH 4) are then determined. The Bernstein test, alternating acid and alkali infusions into the oesophagus, may also be used as an index of mucosal sensitivity to an acid infusion. In addition, an ultrasound scan of the gallbladder should be performed.

The treatment of gastro-oesophageal reflux remains controversial, but should firstly be by medical means. The patient should be advised to lose weight and to avoid excessive stooping and the lifting of heavy weights. He should also be advised to elevate the head of the bed by approximately 6 inches, using wooden blocks for this purpose. Weight reduction alone may produce a dramatic improvement in the patient who suffers mild symptoms of reflux oesophagitis. Abstaining from smoking and reducing alcohol intake are also beneficial.

It is usual to recommend drug therapy in the form of an H_2-receptor antagonist and either metoclopramide or domperidone. The former drug acts by lowering acid output which reduces the effects of the refluxed fluid on the oesophageal mucosa; the latter drugs, by increasing oesophageal and gastric motility, improve clearance of refluxed material and possibly also diminish the volume of the refluxing fluid. Conventional antacids or alginates (e.g. Gaviscon® and Gastrocote®) which form an oil-immiscible antacid layer within the stomach, often produce symptomatic relief.

The principal indication for surgical treatment is failure of conservative therapy. This may be interpreted in different ways by different surgeons, but should oesophageal stricture develop then this is an absolute indication for operative treatment. The severity of oesophagitis *per se* does not accurately predict the need for surgical treatment, nor does the presence of hiatus hernia, unless large. Large hiatus herniae of either a sliding or a rolling nature, however, require surgical treatment; this is because they take up valuable space in the patient's chest (thus compromising cardio-respiratory functions) and may undergo volvulus.

The choice of surgical operation remains controversial, the major aim being to create an intra-abdominal oesophagus. In the 1950s Allison designed a procedure to produce anatomical correction of the hernia and to prevent reflux. The hiatus hernia was reduced, the intra-abdominal length of oesophagus restored and the hiatal crura were repaired around the oesophagus. Although correction of the hiatus hernia was satisfactory, symptomatic reflux was not adequately controlled in a large number of cases; thus the operation is now rarely performed.

Hill's posterior gastropexy was initially designed as a method of fixing the stomach to the posterior abdominal wall, a partial fundoplication was later added. The results are superior to those associated with the Allison repair.

The most commonly performed operation is now the Nissen fundoplication which should be performed using an abdominal approach. Anterior and posterior folds of gastric fundus are wrapped around the lower oesophagus to produce a complete fundoplication. This complete 'wrap around' is efficient in terms of preventing reflux but may be associated with disabling symptoms of 'gas bloat'. A further technique described by Belsey (Mark IV) is performed using a transthoracic approach. The hernia is reduced and a partial fundoplication is performed, fixing the gastric fundus to the oesophagus and returning it into the abdomen.

A totally new approach to the problem is that described by Angelchik. A 'C' shaped silicone cuff is tied around the lower oesophagus where it loosely lies like a horse's halter. The device is effective in preventing reflux in the majority of cases but problems have been reported, in particular persistent dysphagia, stricture formation and erosion into the gastric lumen.

There is still scope for the development of an effective operation for the prevention of gastro-oesophageal reflux.

Case 4

A 78-year-old man presented with a feeling of vague epigastric discomfort and a sensation of regurgitation of food into the lower oesophagus. He was otherwise well, and emphatically denied a history of dysphagia. There was neither a previous history of dyspepsia nor of oesophageal problems. Barium swallow showed a little irregularity at the lower end of the oesophagus, in keeping with reflux oesophagitis. Endoscopy was performed and revealed a slight irregularity of the lower oesophagus which was erythematous. Biopsy of the mucosa showed chronic inflammation only and the patient was treated with cimetidine and metoclopramide. His symptoms initially improved, but 2 months later his trouble recurred, although once again he emphatically denied a history of dysphagia. The investigations were repeated and again biopsy and brush cytology of the lower oesophagus revealed chronic inflammatory cells only. The surgeon remained unhappy with his diagnosis and repeated the investigations 1 month later, when medical therapy had remained unsuccessful. On this occasion a diagnosis of adenocarcinoma was made.

Questions

Why are the results of treating oesophageal neoplasms so poor?

How should the patient be treated?

How should the anastomosis be performed?

Discussion

The problem identified by this case is that, in order to cure oesophageal cancer, the diagnosis must be made at an early stage of the disease; however, confirming the diagnosis under such circumstances can be difficult. Survival in patients with oesophageal cancer is very poor, most patients having disease too advanced for surgical cure at the time of detection. In this case, the histological diagnosis of adeno-carcinoma indicates that the tumour has arisen either in the stomach or in oesophageal mucosa which has undergone prior metaplastic change (Barrett's oesophagus). The pre-sence of such a tumour at the gastro-oesophageal junction is likely to interfere with the competence and continence at that junction, thus predisposing the patient to reflux oeso-phagitis. The problem then becomes one of 'sampling', in that the biopsy is as likely to reveal chronic inflammatory tissue as to indicate the more sinister underlying pathology.

In deciding upon the most appropriate treatment several factors should be considered: (i) the extent of the tumour; (ii) the patient's general condition; (iii) whether complete excision of the tumour is possible; (iv) whether palliation is either feasible or appropriate.

The extent of the tumour can be determined by a combi-nation of endoscopy, chest X-ray, ultrasound of the liver and computerised tomography (CT) of the oesophagus and mediastinum. Endoscopy allows the surgeon to measure the extent and distance of the tumour from the patient's mouth. Submucosal tumour spread may occur for distances of up to 6 cm proximal to the macroscopically obvious edge of the tumour, and this must be taken into account when the sur-geon is deciding upon his strategy for resection. The gen-eral condition of the patient is a major consideration in deciding whether or not to perform oesophagectomy, since those with severe cardiorespiratory problems are unlikely to survive the major trauma involved in performing this type of surgery. Chest X-ray and pulmonary function tests should be performed; the presence of pulmonary metastases would obviate the need for oesophageal resection. The presence of liver metastases on an ultrasound scan of the liver would also exclude the feasibility of curative tumour resection. Computerised tomography (CT) of the lower oesophagus and mediastinum is also useful in assessing the degree of local invasion from the tumour.

The fundamental aims in the treatment of carcinoma of the oesophagus are: either (i) to excise in total the carcinoma and to re-establish oesophageal continuity with the rest of the gastrointestinal tract or (ii) where palliation alone is possible, to treat dysphagia.

The surgical approach and the extent of resection depends upon the anatomical site of the tumour. In view of this, tumours are conveniently divided into those arising from the upper, the middle, and the lower third of the oesophagus. Tumours of the cardio-oesophageal junction and lower third of the oesophagus are commonly approached through a left thoraco-abdominal incision and, after block dissection of the spleen, stomach and lower third of the oesophagus, the oesophagus is replaced. This is performed either by a direct anastomosis of the divided oesophagus to the remaining antrum or by oesophago-jejunal anastomosis (Roux-en-Y method), or by the method described by Ivor Lewis. The latter involves a 2-stage resection, the stomach being mobilised through an upper midline incision, the thoracic part of the operation then being performed through a conventional right thoracotomy. Better access to the oesophagus is achieved using this approach, and mobilization may be easily carried out up to the level of the azygos arch or above, thus ensuring complete local clearance of tumour.

Great care must be exercised in performing the oesophageal anastomosis. The oesophagus is thin-walled and has a relatively poor blood supply; therefore unless meticulous attention is paid to detail, anastomotic dehiscence can occur with a high incidence of fatality. The author prefers to use 2 layers of suture material; for the inner layer which is most likely to slough, interrupted sutures are preferable to continuous ones. Continuous sutures are very suitable for the outer layer of the anastomosis. The sutures should not be tied so tightly as to interfere with the blood supply at the anastomosis. The 2 factors which most commonly precipitate an anastomotic dehiscence are ischaemia and surrounding infection; these lead to oedema and the cutting out from tissues of anastomotic sutures.

The only form of palliation likely to benefit the above patient is oesophageal intubation; neither radiotherapy nor chemotherapy have a role in the treatment of an adenocarcinoma of the gastro-oesophageal junction. Intubation can be performed either operatively or endoscopically. Mousseau-Barbin or Celestin tubes are used for tumours of the middle and lower third of the oesophagus. Prior to insertion, the oesophagus requires dilatation; this may be performed either preoperatively and endoscopically or, at the time of operation, through the stomach. Gum elastic bougies are passed along the stomach and through the oesophageal stricture and into the mouth where they may be attached to the Celestin tube which is then railroaded through the stricture. The funnel of the tube lies above the stricture, its cylindrical portion is divided at the level of the mid-stomach and the lower end is attached to the gastric wall to prevent proximal migration.

A simple, but useful, technique when inserting these tubes is the use of a fine nylon line with some small lead weights attached to one end. On the evening prior to surgery the patient is requested to swallow the weights, and sufficient line is allowed to pass into the oesophagus to permit passage of the weights into the gastric antrum. The proximal end of the line is then firmly strapped to the side of the patient's face. Despite the presence of a tight oesophageal stricture, it is usual for the small weights to migrate through the stricture overnight; thus an X-ray taken the following morning will usually show the weights in the patient's stomach. The intragastric line can then be retrieved through a small gastrotomy, and may be used to pull the tube through and across the stricture.

The Nottingham tube is an innovative device which can be inserted using an endoscopic technique. An end-viewing gastroscope is passed into the oesophagus as far as the stricture, and a fine wire is passed through the endoscope and the stricture. The stricture is then dilated using Celestin graded dilators and finally the Nottingham tube is passed over the guide wire on an introducer. When placed inside the stricture, the introducer is removed leaving the stricture intubated. A liquid diet can then be taken by the patient. Postoperative care should be taken to prevent aspiration and food bolus obstruction.

Case 5

A 55-year-old man presented with an 8-month history of epigastric pain starting approximately 45 minutes after a meal. This pain persisted for between 30-60 minutes, although bouts of pain were sometimes irregular and unrelated to food. There was no history of nocturnal pain and abstinence from food tended to be associated with absence of pain. In recent months, there had been radiation of pain to the patient's back and concomitant anorexia with the loss of half a stone in weight. The dyspeptic attacks had been episodic, having been particularly severe over the month prior to presentation. The patient worked on the shop floor in the motor industry. He smoked 40 cigarettes/day and drank 20 pints of beer/week. There was no past medical history of note and no history of peptic ulceration.

On examination the only abnormality was some rather diffuse epigastric tenderness but no guarding and no abdominal masses.

Questions

How should this patient be investigated?
How should the patient be treated?

Discussion

The major differential diagnosis here lies between a peptic ulcer, a gastric cancer and a pancreatic cancer. Other possibilities relate chiefly to biliary tract disorders, in particular cholelithiasis, or possibly a hepato-biliary neoplasm. The most appropriate initial investigation is an upper gastrointestinal endoscopy, which, in this case, revealed a lesser curve gastric ulcer. Full blood count and chest X-ray should also be performed. A barium meal can be a useful adjunct to endoscopy when gastric pathology has been identified on the former examination. Most gastric ulcers are quite easily identified on endoscopy, where multiple biopsies should be taken from the ulcer edge to exclude malignancy.

The management of peptic ulcer has markedly changed

in recent years following the advent of both endoscopy, which has added to our understanding of the natural history, and the H_2-receptor antagonists. Before treating a gastric ulcer it is of fundamental importance to exclude any possibility of malignancy within the ulcer. Medical management is then indicated, in the first place. Spices, excess tea, coffee and alcoholic beverages should be avoided. The patient should also be advised to stop smoking. Anti-inflammatory drugs should be stopped or replaced by enterically coated substitutes where these are necessary. H_2-receptor antagonists (e.g. cimetidine or ranitidine) form the mainstay of current medical management and, after a 6-week course, over 80% of gastric ulcers will have completely healed. The endoscopy should be repeated after the 6-week course of the H_2-receptor antagonist. The duration of treatment remains controversial but, following its cessation, relapse rates are high. In view of this, some clinicians employ long-term maintenance therapy with a low-dose nocturnally administered H_2-receptor antagonist; despite this, an appreciable number will still relapse. Other drugs, in particular carbenoxolone sodium, sucralfate and DeNol, have been shown to be effective in healing gastric ulcers.

The indications for surgery in gastric ulcer are: (i) failure of medical treatment; (ii) repeated relapse following successful medical treatment and (iii) the possibility of malignant change in the ulcer. The operation of choice is a Billroth I gastrectomy in which the ulcer is excised along with the distal stomach, and then a gastro-duodenal anastomosis is subsequently performed. Results following this operation are generally very good; recurrent ulceration is uncommon (2%) and the operative mortality is approximately 1%. Various forms of vagotomy, including highly-selective forms, have been recommended for gastric ulcer; however, the results are probably inferior to those following Billroth I gastrectomy. Gastric ulcers situated high on the lesser curvature of the stomach may pose particular problems at operation. The basic operative treatment remains a Billroth I gastrectomy but, in addition, a sliver of lesser curvature almost up to the oesophago-gastric junction, and including the ulcer, is excised. This manoeuvre is referred to as the Pauchet procedure. Prepyloric gastric ulcers and gastric ulcers secondary to duodenal ulcers should be treated as duodenal ulcers.

Case 6

A 38-year-old man first presented with a small haematemesis and a 5-year history of intermittent epigastric pain, which had been particularly severe for 4 days prior to presentation. Endoscopy at this stage showed a distal oesophagitis, antral gastritis and duodenitis; however, no obvious source of bleeding was seen and there was no evidence of a chronic duodenal ulcer. The patient was treated with a one month course of cimetidine (1 g/day) and his symptoms rapidly settled.

Two years later he again presented with severe dyspepsia of 6 months duration and was shown to have a prepyloric gastric ulcer. He was treated with Cimetidine (1 g/day) for 2 months and then advised to take 400 mg at night, which he continued to take, albeit intermittently. Nine months after the diagnosis of his ulcer the patient presented as an emergency with the sudden onset of severe epigastric pain, but no previous dyspepsia. He was pale and shocked with a rigid upper abdomen. Plain abdominal X-ray showed the presence of free gas under the diaphragm. At laparotomy, the prepyloric gastric ulcer had perforated through the posterior aspect of the lesser curvature into the lesser sac; in addition, a generalised peritonitis was present with 1300 ml of fluid in the peritoneal cavity.

Questions

What is the surgical treatment of choice?

Discussion

Faced with a perforated prepyloric gastric ulcer, the surgical treatment of choice depends upon the patient's condition and the experience of the surgeon performing the emergency procedure. If unable to acquire the help of a more senior colleague, the junior surgeon may simply oversew the perforation. Such a policy is highly likely to be temporary in its effect as the patient would be markedly prone to recurrent ulceration. However, this procedure in the emergency situation would be life-saving, and safe, simple and quick to perform. The more experienced surgeon should perform an acid reducing operation in addition to oversewing or excising the perforated area. The choice of acid-reducing procedure lies between truncal vagotomy and pyloroplasty (with oversew), highly selective vagotomy or truncal vagotomy with antrectomy. There is a small risk of malignancy in patients with gastric ulcer; vagotomy and pyloroplasty therefore should not be performed without an accompanying excision of the ulcerated area. Highly selective vagotomy has been shown to be particularly unsatisfactory for prepyloric ulcer, as regards a high incidence of recurrence; it is also difficult and time-consuming to perform in the presence of peritonitis from perforation.

Truncal vagotomy and antrectomy combined is, in the author's opinion, the treatment of choice. It is the most effective acid-inhibiting operation, allowing excision of the ulcer and the ulcer-bearing gastrin-secreting areas of the stomach. Vagotomy alone results in a sixty five per cent reduction in acid output, antrectomy likewise; together they produce over a ninety per cent inhibition of acid output and a low risk of recurrent ulcer.

The factors against performing truncal vagotomy in combination with antrectomy are that it is a more major procedure and thus carries a higher mortality and morbidity. The short-term morbidity relates to septic complications, the long-term to dumping, diarrhoea, distension and duodenogastric reflux.

A further point of discussion relating to this case is that perforation occurred whilst the patient was taking an H_2-receptor blocker for maintenance treatment. Approximately 35 per cent of ulcers will recur over a one-year period on nocturnal maintenance therapy, and there is no evidence that H_2-receptor blockers have influenced the incidence of perforated peptic ulcer. The fall in incidence of peptic ulceration preceded the introduction of these drugs in 1977. Indeed, in recent years, there has again been a slight rise in the incidence of perforated ulcers, particularly in elderly females taking non-steroidal anti-inflammatory drugs.

The patient underwent truncal vagotomy with antrectomy, made a good postoperative recovery and has remained well to date. The incidence of recurrent ulcer formation after this operation is of the order of 2%.

Case 7

A 42-year-old woman had a 10-year history of duodenal ulcer. In recent years this had become more troublesome, recurring repeatedly after completion of courses of cimetidine and, occasionally, whilst taking the drug. An active ulcer was demonstrated on endoscopy, and had been shown on 2 barium meals performed over several previous years. In view of the persistence of her symptoms and problems with drug compliance, a decision was made to perform elective surgery. A truncal vagotomy and pyloroplasty was carried out and the patient made a satisfactory recovery in terms of abatement of her ulcer pain but developed mild diarrhoea. This was particularly troublesome in the early morning and whilst episodic, tended to be heralded by post-prandial colicky lower abdominal pain. The diarrhoea was watery and had, very occasionally, led to incontinence which the patient had been reluctant to admit except on direct questioning.

Over an 18-month period the diarrhoea spontaneously improved to the extent of becoming no longer troublesome. However, right hypochondrial pain had developed over recent months and had been particularly severe on 2 occasions. Both these exacerbations had occurred in the evening, following on after eating a heavy and particularly fatty meal. The pain, which was colicky in nature, spread across the upper abdomen and radiated posteriorly into the interscapular region. On each occasion it was associated with vomiting for about 8 hours. There was no history of jaundice. Upper gastrointestinal endoscopy showed no abnormality, but an ultrasound scan of the upper abdomen revealed two gallstones, biliary debris and a thick-walled gallbladder. A cholecystectomy was then performed. Postoperatively, the patient developed severe diarrhoea and an epigastric burning sensation. The diarrhoea was more severe than in the early stages after the vagotomy and pyloroplasty, but was still episodic and associated with bouts of incontinence. The epigastric pain was continuously present, often worse at night and when the stomach was empty. Vomiting was uncommon, but tended to be stained with bile and of small volume.

Questions

What is the pathogenesis of this patient's problem?
What treatment is available?

Discussion

The combination of truncal vagotomy with drainage together with cholecystectomy is prone to produce several undesirable sequelae, referred to as the postvagotomy and cholecystectomy syndrome. This consists of a combination of diarrhoea and bile reflux gastritis. A cholecystectomy performed after a previous vagotomy and drainage procedure can produce diarrhoea and reflux gastritis not present following the vagotomy alone. The mechanism relates to the mechanical handling of bile acids by the small intestine and duodenum. Following cholecystectomy, bile continuously trickles into the duodenum and small bowel; therefore when the stomach is empty, bile is freer to reflux through the incompetent gastric outlet thus producing gastritis. After a meal, increased peristalsis dumps the bile, which had been lying in the small bowel lumen, onto the colonic mucosa where it produces diarrhoea by the outpouring of electrolytes.

The problem is difficult to treat. Bile acid binding agents such as aluminium hydroxide and cholestyramine have proved disappointing in the treatment of bile reflux gastritis, as has sucralfate. These substances, particularly cholestyramine, are more effective in treating the diarrhoea; however, this agent is unpalatable and, in view of the episodic nature of the symptoms, patient compliance is not consistently good. Biliary diversion by Roux-en-Y anastomosis using a 50 cm interposition is effective in preventing bile from reaching the stomach. An antrectomy should be carried out in addition to this procedure. The operation is often also effective in improving the diarrhoea; this it achieves by slowing down intestinal transit time and providing a loop of duodenum and small intestine, lying outside the main stream of the gastrointestinal tract, in which bile can accumulate without being hurried through onto the colonic mucosa. The patients' symptoms are often disabling and of sufficient severity to warrant this operative procedure.

Case 8

A 49-year-old man presented with a 4-month history of dyspeptic symptoms. He complained of epigastric pain which occurred about 1 hour after meals lasting for up to 2 hours and was aggravated by spices and alcohol. The only relieving factor was abstinence from food. The patient had lost 3/4 stone in weight during the course of his illness, and felt lethargic and easily fatigued. Over the 2- to 3-week period prior to presentation he had become anorexic. On examination there were no abnormalities. The patient was, however, mildly anaemic, with a haemoglobin of 11g/dl.

Questions

How should this patient be investigated?
What is the differential diagnosis?
What is the appropriate treatment?

Discussion

The combination of 'anorexia, anaemia and asthenia' must always be taken very seriously, and is suggestive of a malignant process, until the diagnosis is proved otherwise. The most likely sites of malignancy giving rise to this group of symptoms are the stomach, the bronchus, the caecum and the pancreas. Malignancies may present directly as a result of manifestations produced by the primary tumour, as a result of the presence of metastasis, or as a result of the nonmetastatic manifestations of a malignant process. The dyspeptic symptoms present in this patient would make carcinoma of the stomach the most likely cause of his problem. The patient should be investigated by full blood count, liver function tests, chest X-ray, barium meal and upper gastrointestinal endoscopy. In this case the full blood count showed the patient to be mildly anaemic with a raised erythrocyte sedimentation rate of 30 mm in the first hour. Liver function tests were entirely normal, as was the chest X-ray. A barium meal showed a large gastric ulcer, high on the lesser curve of the stomach with prominent rolled edges. Upper gastrointestinal tract endoscopy confirmed the presence of a large ulcer, and multiple biopsies were taken from the ulcer crater and the edge of the ulcerated area. In addition, there was a mild gastritis present in the body of the stomach. The biopsies confirmed the diagnosis of adenocarcinoma of the stomach and an ultrasound scan of the liver was performed, the results of which were entirely within normal limits.

There were no known predisposing factors to carcinoma of the stomach in this patient. He did not have pernicious anaemia and had not previously undergone gastric surgery. There was no family history of gastric cancer, and the history of dyspepsia was relatively recent. It is possible that the carcinoma arose in pre-existing benign gastric ulcer, although whether the ulcer preceded the cancer or vice versa is debatable. There can, however, be little doubt that about 2% of gastric cancers arise in pre-existing benign gastric ulcers. The patient smoked 20 cigarettes/day and worked as a painter. Smoking and certain occupations, of which painting is one, have been associated with an increased incidence of gastric malignancy. At this stage in the investigation the major unknown factors relating ultimately to the prognosis of this tumour are the depth of invasion of the tumour, the degree of lymphatic involvement, the evidence of blood spread or of transcoelomic deposits of malignant disease. It is possible that computerised tomography might give the surgeon more information regarding these parameters, but not all centres have access to this mode of investigation, and those which do are often so heavily committed to other programmes of investigation that the staging of gastric cancer is a low priority. Equally, the evidence that computerised tomography is accurate in demonstrating the extent of malignancy is wanting.

The curative potential of surgical treatment is dependent upon the depth of invasion of the stomach wall by the cancer and the presence or absence of lymph node metastasis or more distant spread. Early gastric cancer, by definition that confined to the mucosa and sub-mucosa, has an extremely good prognosis with over 90% being alive at 5 years. But advanced gastric cancer has a 5-year survival rate of less than 10%. The presence of lymph node involvement dramatically reduces the 5-year survival rate, and for those with more distant spread to liver, lung or brain, the 5-year survival rate is practically zero. Surgery provides the only possibility of a cure in gastric cancer. Even so 'curative resection' can only be offered to less than half the patients at the time of presentation, and the major problem facing the clinician in the treatment of gastric cancer is that the condition usually presents at an advanced stage as conversely, early gastric cancer is frequently totally asymptomatic. Laparotomy remains not only the mainstay of treatment, but provides an accurate assessment of the extent of the spread of the disorder. In addition, if curative resection is impossible, it is often feasible to improve the quality of the patient's life by some form of palliative surgery.

At operation, this patient was found to have a 5 cm by 3 cm tumour on the lesser curvature of the stomach with a solitary involved lymph node, close to the lesser curvature along the left gastric veins. There was neither evidence of invasion into the pancreas, the under surface of the liver, nor of transperitoneal spread. Equally there was no evidence of blood spread. Clearly this was a case of advanced gastric cancer, but one which was amenable to potentially curative surgery.

With regard to the operative classification of lymph node involvement, the Japanese Research Society for Gastric Cancer have designated four tiers of lymph node involvement, that is N1 to N4. N1 nodes are those immediately surrounding the stomach. N2 nodes are those around the left gastric, common hepatic, splenic and coeliac arteries. Lymph nodes designated N3 are those in the hepato-duodenal ligament, posterior part of the pancreas, root of the mesentery and the para-oesophageal region. Any more distant lymph nodes than these are designated N4. The categories N1 to N4 indicate progressive advancement of the disease and correlate with the ultimate survival which decreases accordingly as more distant lymph nodes are involved.

The aims of surgical treatment must be to excise *in toto* the primary tumour and any associated lymph node involvement. The Japanese have shown improved results of surgery with more radical resection and have defined the extent of gastrectomy as R1, R2 or R3 according to the extent of the lymphadenectomy.

The most frequent site of recurrent disease following partial gastrectomy for gastric cancer is in the gastric stump; this has led surgeons in recent years to prefer total gastrectomy. However, this is only justifiable in the best surgical hands when the mortality associated with total gastrectomy is sufficiently low so as not to preclude the potential benefit gained from the more radical resection. Regrettably, the first reports on total gastrectomy all showed that the increased operative mortality outweighed the potential overall benefits of the more radical operation. However, the Japanese have recently reported a postoperative mortality of only 3.7% which would appear to justify the more radical surgical approach.

This patient was treated by total gastrectomy. The tumour was high on the lesser curvature and it would not have been safe to leave a small cuff of gastric remnant below the oesophago-gastric junction. A 2-layer oesophago-jejunal anastomosis was performed end-to-side and an enteroanastomosis was then carried out 10 cm distal to this to obviate bile reflux into the lower oesophagus and to create something of a reservoir for food. The patient made an uneventful postoperative recovery and histological examination of the resected specimen showed lymph node involvement of the perigastric and left gastric nodes but no spread beyond this. The patient has remained well for a period of 2 years following his resection.

Case 9

A 55-year-old man sustained an inferior myocardial infarction, followed by a second ischaemic episode some nine months later. He then presented with an iron-deficiency anaemia which exacerbated his angina pectoris. The patient had begun to feel weak and was breathless on minor exertion. Faecal occult blood estimations were repeatedly positive. His haemoglobin concentration was 8g/dl, MCV 7.7 pg, MCH 26.7 pg and MCHC 30.5g/dl. Chest X-ray was normal. A barium meal showed a gross deformity of the anterior gastric wall extending along the proximal half of the greater curvature. There was a central crater with radiating coarse folds. The edges of the lesion showed marked shouldering. The features were those of a gastric neoplasm. Gastroscopy was performed with biopsy from six sites within and on the edge of the ulcerated mass. These small biopsies showed gastric mucosa with a mixed acute and chronic inflammatory cell infiltrate; there was no evidence of malignancy.

Questions

What treatment is indicated?
Should the patient have received any further therapy?

Discussion

A laparotomy was performed and revealed a large gastric ulcer in the proximal stomach. There was no associated lymphadenopathy. A biopsy of the lesion was submitted for frozen section and reported as a gastric lymphoma. Total gastrectomy was carried out with an oesophago-jejunal anastomosis and an enteroanastomosis. The greater and lesser omenta were excised *in toto*.

The patient made an uneventful postoperative recovery. Six months after his gastrectomy the patient's angina became more troublesome and he underwent coronary artery bypass surgery from which he made an uneventful recovery and has remained well with no evidence of recurrence of his lymphoma.

The surgical treatment of gastric lymphoma should be identical to that of gastric cancer. Surgical treatment alone yields a 5-year survival rate of the order of 33%. Total gastrectomy is indicated in all cases except those where the tumour is early and entirely confined to a relatively small area of the distal stomach, when subtotal gastrectomy is carried out. In some cases, it is difficult to distinguish a true lymphoma from the so-called 'pseudolymphoma' of the stomach. Prognosis is directly proportional to the extent of lymph node involvement, and is better for the lymphocytic than the histiocytic variety. In this patient surgical excision appeared to have been complete; there was no lymph node involvement and the patient also suffered from myocardial ischaemia and was awaiting coronary artery bypass surgery. When radiation therapy is used it is administered in a dose of 4000 to 5000 rads (cGy), given in 20 to 25 fractions. Total abdominal irradiation is applied, with additional boosting doses directed at the stomach bed, para-aortic, splenic, *porta hepatis* and pancreatico-duodenal areas. Using high dose radiation as an adjunct to surgery, the five year survival in the Sloan-Kettering study was 85%. A role for chemotherapy as an adjunct to surgery has not been established.

Case 10

A 42-year-old woman presented with a 2-day history of abdominal pain associated with vomiting. Over the previous 2 years she had experienced vague upper abdominal pains which were related to the ingestion of fatty foods. The pain she was suffering at the present time had come on gradually during the day becoming colicky in nature with maximal discomfort in the right upper quadrant of the abdomen and radiation through to the back. There was no history of haematemesis or melaena and her appetite and weight had been steady.

On examination, she was pyrexial with a temperature of 39.9°C. Her blood pressure was normal, but she had a pronounced tachycardia of 120 beats/min. There was no evidence of jaundice or anaemia. Examination of the abdomen confirmed that she was very tender in the right upper quadrant, with evidence of rebound tenderness and localised peritonitis. A positive Murphy's sign was also present. The rest of the abdomen appeared normal.

Investigations

Full blood count: Hb 13.6 g/dl, white cell count 16.4 × 10 g/l, urea and electrolytes normal, amylase 160 U/l, alkaline phosphatase 180 U/l, bilirubin 32 µmol/l, ALT 65 U/l. Urinalysis was negative. Chest X-ray was normal. Abdominal X-ray showed no specific abnormality.

Questions

What is the differential diagnosis in this patient and how could the eventual diagnosis be confirmed?
Describe the management of this patient?

Discussion

Although this patient presents a typical history of acute cholecystitis, the diagnosis is often not quite so clear. A perforated duodenal ulcer must be excluded by means of abdominal and chest X-ray and a gastrograffin swallow may be needed to confirm this diagnosis. An acute duodenal ulcer may also present with a similar pain which should be excluded by gastroscopy. Acute pancreatitis can, in most cases, be excluded by the presence of a normal serum amylase. The presence of pyelonephritis must be tested by means of urinalysis and MSU testing. Occasionally a high retrocaecal appendix may occur with pain in a similar area. Right-sided chest conditions such as pulmonary embolism and right lower lobe pneumonia may also be confused with cholecystitis and the possibility of these should be excluded by means of clinical examination and chest X-ray.

Often, the only abnormalities found on blood testing in a patient with acute cholecystitis are those of a slightly raised white count and minimally deranged liver function tests. Should frank jaundice be present, then the suspicion of a stone in the common bile duct must be considered.

The diagnosis should always be confirmed by means of ultrasonography. The advent of the new ultrasound machines has enabled accuracy rates of above 90% to be achieved in most centres. The presence of a normal ultrasound with the gallbladder clearly visualised should virtually rule out the possibility of acute cholecystitis. The recent use of HIDA scanning, whereby an isotope is injected intravenously and selectively excreted into bile, has shown promising results in that the presence of acute cholecystitis is confirmed by the absence of uptake by the gallbladder following injection. Once the acute inflammation has settled an oral cholecystogram may be performed; this will show either the presence of a non-functioning gallbladder or multiple gallstones within the gallbladder. A plain abdominal X-ray is rarely of help in acute cholecystitis since stones are only visible in 10–15% of cases. In the presence of jaundice, an ultrasound scan will show the presence of dilated bile ducts, and the presence of a stone causing jaundice may be confirmed on PTC examination or by ERCP.

The initial management of this patient consisted of intravenous fluid replacement and the stopping of oral fluid intake. In cases where vomiting is present a nasogastric tube may need to be passed. Analgesia is given in the form of intramuscular pethidine, and frequently antiemetics, (e.g. metoclopramide) may be required.

As acute cholecystitis is related to the presence of infection within the gallbladder and biliary tree, there is little doubt that parenterally administered antibiotics have an important part to play in the management of these patients. The choice of antibiotics must depend upon the organisms likely to be present and the degree of penetration of antibiotics into the bile. Most infections are caused by aerobic coliform organisms and occasionally *Streptococcus faecalis.* Anaerobic organisms are, however, increasingly recognised as being of importance in the inflammatory process. A variety of antibiotics may be used to treat these patients and these include cephalosporins, cotrimoxazole and aminoglycosides. Metronidazole should also be given to these patients.

This patient was managed with an intravenous cephalosporin and metronidazole suppositories. With this treatment her condition recovered rapidly and her temperature fell to normal.

A proportion of patients, however, fail to settle down completely on this management and, in these, the diagnosis is likely to be that of empyema of the gallbladder. These patients, once the diagnosis is confirmed with ultrasonography, require urgent cholecystectomy.

Currently there is much controversy as to whether operation in patients with acute cholecystitis should be carried out in the early phase of the disorder or at a later date. Most centres perform urgent cholecystectomy, within one to two days of admission, when the diagnosis has been confirmed by ultrasonography or HIDA scanning. The advantages of an early cholecystectomy performed as a semi-elective procedure are that (i) the patient requires only one admission and (ii) in those patients who are sent home prior to a late operation there is a high incidence of recurrence with complications. Indeed, 20% of patients with acute cholecystitis who are sent home for a later operation have another emergency admission before their elective admission. Surgery performed within the first four days is relatively straightforward as there is much oedema around the gallbladder which may facilitate dissection. All patients should have a cholecystectomy performed and operative cholangiography is mandatory to exclude the possibility of common bile duct stones. Prophylactic antibiotic cover should be used in all patients. In patients where diagnosis is uncertain they should be allowed to settle down and then be discharged. An oral cholecystogram, or a repeat ultrasound examination, is carried out after discharge from hospital. These patients should then be re-admitted, within 2 months, for elective cholecystectomy. Recent studies have shown little evidence of increased mortality following 'emergency surgery'. In the acute operative phase there is an increase in biliary infection and twice the incidence of choledocholithiasis. In some patients, dissection may be extremely difficult due to severe infection with small abcesses being present around the gallbladder. These cases require broad-spectrum antibiotic prophylaxis, an experienced surgeon and, as already emphasised, operative cholangiography must be carried out in all.

An ultrasound scan was performed on this patient within 48 hours of admission. This revealed the presence of multiple stones within the gallbladder. A cholecystectomy was subsequently performed on the next operative list, and operative cholangiography was normal. This patient's drain was removed 3 days postoperatively, and she made an excellent recovery with no septic complications.

Case 11

A 62-year-old woman presented with a 2-week history of upper abdominal pain which was colicky in nature and radiated posteriorly. Over the past week she had become markedly jaundiced, passing pale, bulky stools and dark urine. She had also developed anorexia and generalised pruritus. On two occasions she had had shivering attacks which resolved spontaneously. In her past history there was a suggestion of fatty food intolerance, but neither history of alcohol abuse nor diabetes.

On examination, she was deeply jaundiced but there were none of the stigmata of liver failure. Her skin showed evidence of scratch marks and she was noticed to be pyrexial with a temperature of 38.5°C. Examination of the abdomen was unremarkable apart from tenderness in the epigastrium and in the right upper quadrant. Rectal examination confirmed the presence of pale stools but no other abnormality was present.

Investigations

Haemoglobin 13.6 G/dl. White cell count $18.9 \times 10^9/l$. Urea and electrolytes normal. Creatinine 130 μmol/l. Bilirubin 250 μmol/l. ALT 110 U/l. Alkaline phosphatase 985 U/l. Prothrombin ratio 1.8:1. Hepatitis B surface antigen negative. Gammaglutamyltranspeptidase normal. Urinalysis was strongly positive for bilirubin.

Questions

What is your differential diagnosis and what investigations are available to confirm this?
How would you manage this patient?

Discussion

The clinical history and liver function tests all suggest the presence of an obstructive jaundice. The short history, pyrexia and a raised white cell count are suggestive of gallstone-induced obstructive jaundice in association with cholangitis. In patients with jaundice it is important to rule out the presence of primary liver disease such as hepatitis, primary biliary cirrhosis and liver failure. Alcoholic liver disease and drug-induced cholestasis must also be excluded.

Metastatic carcinoma of the liver can result in jaundice which is extremely difficult to differentiate from obstructive jaundice. Obstructive jaundice itself may be related to the presence of a gallstone in the common bile duct or obstruction by malignancy, such as carcinoma of the pancreas, cholangiocarcinoma and secondary tumour within lymph nodes at the *porta hepatis*. After the initial blood tests are performed the investigation of choice is ultrasonography. This will differentiate the presence of obstructive jaundice, with dilated intra- and extra-hepatic ducts, from primary liver disease, where no dilated ducts are seen.

The accuracy of this differentiation should be above 95% in experienced hands. Stones themselves may be seen within the gallbladder, although these are less easily identified within the common bile duct because of the presence of overlying bowel gas.

If the ultrasound scan shows no evidence of dilated ducts the patient should be further investigated medically. Liver function tests should be repeated and the patient will require liver biopsy either performed percutaneously or via a laparoscope. Before proceeding to liver biopsy the prothrombin time must be normal or corrected by administration of vitamin K.

Further investigation of the patient with dilated ducts may require the use of invasive procedures. Therefore the patient should be given intravenous antibiotics which should include an aminoglycoside (e.g. gentamycin) or a cephalosporin (e.g. cefoxitin). The patient should also be started on intramuscular vitamin K in an attempt to correct prolonged clotting times, as haemorrhage can be a serious complication in these patients.

The two main investigative techniques available are: (i) percutaneous transhepatic cholangiography (PTC) and (ii) endoscopic retrograde cholangiopancreatography. With PTC a skinny Chiba needle is passed through the liver into the dilated bile duct and dye injected into the biliary tree. Using this method the site and nature of the obstruction may be easily identified. PTC is an investigation that has been associated with several complications such as bile leak, or biliary peritonitis, haemorrhage and septicaemia. The incidence of these complications should, however, be minimal if the previously mentioned precautions are taken. In patients with severe cholangitis and marked obstructive jaundice, a drainage catheter may be inserted into the dilated biliary tree at the time of PTC examination. This allows a preoperative period of biliary decompression, and potentially, the control of sepsis before operation is carried out. At present, controversy exists as to whether preoperative biliary decompression is beneficial, since the problems of catheter management, particularly those of a septic nature, can be very serious.

The other main investigative technique used is that of endoscopic retrograde cholangiopancreatography (ERCP). A side-viewing flexible endoscope is passed into the duodenum and the ampulla of Vater cannulated. Dye is injected into both the pancreatic and biliary trees. The presence or absence of obstruction in the biliary tree is easily identified and in those patients with a stone blocking the common bile duct an endoscopic sphincterotomy may also be carried out. The same precautions as previously mentioned for PTC are mandatory. The sphincterotomy can be performed with a special cutting papillotome and the stones themselves can either be allowed to fall out or are pulled through the ampulla by means of a Dormia basket. Therefore in experienced hands ERCP may be the investigation of choice since this allows a corrective procedure to be carried out at the same time. Following recovery, the gallbladder should be removed at operation.

Computerised tomography (CT) has been advocated in the management of patients with obstructive jaundice. This investigation will certainly allow better visualisation of the pancreas and is non-invasive.

Laparoscopy is also used by some surgeons since liver biopsy can be carried out at the same time and direct cholangiography performed by transhepatic needle puncture of the gallbladder under direct vision.

In this patient, ultrasonography confirmed the presence of dilated bile ducts with stones present within the gallbladder. A percutaneous transhepatic cholangiogram was performed which showed the presence of two stones at the lower end of the common bile duct. The bile duct itself was grossly dilated having a diameter of 3 cm. The patient was prepared for theatre with intravenous antibiotics and intramuscular vitamin K. For 24 hours preoperatively, she was given intravenous fluids (1 litre, 8-hourly). A urethral catheter was also passed. It is very important to establish a good urine output in these patients to avoid postoperative renal failure which is related to the presence of endotoxins and is often fatal. In patients where diuresis is poor, mannitol should be given in the immediate preoperative phase and peroperatively.

At operation, the gallbladder was inflamed and contained several stones. An operative cholangiogram confirmed the findings of the PTC examination. The common bile duct was dilated and was explored. Two large stones were present at its lower end, one of which could be removed easily. The other stone was firmly impacted and could not be removed. In this situation the surgeon is faced with two alternatives. Firstly and particularly in the severely ill patient, a simple choledochoduodenostomy could be performed, this will relieve the patient of her jaundice but will, however, leave the stone in place with its attendant morbidity. In this patient, the duodenum was opened and a sphincterotomy performed; this allowed the gallstone to be easily removed. The edges of the common bile duct were then sutured to the duodenal mucosa forming a sphincteroplasty. A choledochoscope was passed along the dilated biliary tree but no further stones could be identified. Choledochoscopy should be used in all such patients as stones can be easily overlooked and left within the intrahepatic biliary radicals. Following this procedure, the bile duct was closed around a T-tube which was left *in situ.*

The duodenum was carefully closed with two layers of catgut; there is small incidence of duodenal fistula and leakage following this procedure. A suction drain was placed in the right upper quadrant of the abdomen in close proximity to the duodenum and the bile duct.

Post-operatively, the patient received intravenous fluids and antibiotics and made a slow and steady recovery. Her jaundice cleared rapidly and she was discharged feeling well, ten days later.

In those patients where a T-tube has been placed, a cholangiogram should be performed through this on the eighth day before the T tube is removed.

There is a significant morbidity and mortality associated with operations in patients with obstructive jaundice. This is related to (i) the presence of sepsis, (ii) uncontrolled bleeding, (iii) subphrenic abscess formation, (iv) renal failure, (v) a high incidence of postoperative gastrointestinal bleeding and (vi) impaired wound healing leading to dehiscence of the abdomen. Careful preoperative management and surgical technique should reduce these dangers to a minimum. Nevertheless the mortality rate is 10-20% in these patients. Several factors have been found to be associated with a high operative risk. These are the presence of severe obstructive jaundice with a bilirubin of greater than 400 µmol/l, marked infection and cholangitis, a low albumin and haematocrit indicating poor nutrition, a high creatinine level, suggesting a degree of renal impairment and the presence of septicaemia.

Case 12

A 26-year-old woman was admitted for an elective cholecystectomy which was performed by a Surgical registrar. On operative cholangiography, the ducts were described as small and normal in appearance. Postoperatively, a biliary fistula developed which discharged approximately 500 ml/day. The fistula had persisted for six weeks and there had been two episodes of jaundice before it spontaneously resolved. Three months later, the patient again became jaundiced and was referred to another centre. On examination, there was a two-finger enlargement of the liver which was tender, no other abnormality was present. The bilirubin concentration was 42µmol/l, alkaline phosphatase 757 U/l, GOT 125 U/l, the total protein was 77 g/l, and the albumin 35 g/l. An ultrasound scan and computerised tomography suggested some enlargement of the pancreatic head but no other abnormality. An isotope scan using the radiopharmaceutical 99 mTc HIDA showed very poor hepatic uptake of the tracer and slow elimination. A small amount of radioactivity was, however, seen in the intestine. Percutaneous transhepatic cholangiography showed a stenosis at the junction of the right and left hepatic ducts with no evidence of contrast material passing beyond this into the lower common bile duct. There was only slight dilatation of the intrahepatic biliary radicles.

Questions

What is the most likely diagnosis?
What treatment is indicated?

Discussion

The patient had a stricture at the junction of the right and left hepatic ducts extending down the common hepatic duct for about 3 cm. This biliary stricture had developed as a result of trauma to the common bile duct at the time of cholecystectomy. Anatomical anomalies in this region make the duct system vulnerable to damage. Also the presence of a very short or absent cystic duct may lead the surgeon to confuse the common bile duct and the cystic duct resulting in the excision of the former. This leaves a large gap between the common hepatic duct and the divided portion of the common bile duct, thus a total biliary fistula ensues. Alternatively the common hepatic duct may be completely ligated, resulting in obstructive jaundice, or the common hepatic and common bile ducts may be tented as a result of traction on the gallblader whereupon a ligature is placed around these either completely or partially occluding the lumen of the bile duct. Bleeding from the cystic artery, thus obscuring the surgeon's view of the duct system, may lead the inexperienced surgeon to place a clamp either partly or completely across the common bile duct, in the hope of arresting haemorrhage.

To prevent duct injury the surgeon must firstly identify, ligate and divide the cystic artery before the cystic duct, and, secondly, identify at least a 2 cm length of the common bile and common hepatic ducts prior to division of the cystic duct. Wherever doubt exists, the gallbladder should be mobilised retrogradely before clamping the cystic duct. If this is not possible a cholecystostomy should be performed; cholecystectomy is then carried out at a later date. The use of operative cholangiography prior to removal of the gallbladder may facilitate identification of the ducts.

Biliary drainage must be promptly re-established; in this case the upper end of the common hepatic duct was divided at the junction of the right and left hepatic ducts. These ducts may be anastomosed either separately, or if possible together, to a loop of jejunum. The usual form of reconstruction is by Roux-en-Y anastomosis, though some prefer a hepaticojejunostomy with an enteroanastomosis. It was possible in this case to bring a Roux loop up to the *porta hepatis* and anastomose this to the confluence of the ducts.

Postoperatively, the patient made a good recovery but 4 years later developed repeated bouts of right hypochondrial pain, jaundice and pyrexia. A percutaneous transhepatic cholangiogram showed a stricture at the junction between the hepatic ducts and the Roux loop. A further exploration was carried out 5 years after the first, the new stricture was excised and the jejunum was mobilised up into the *porta hepatis* using the mucosal graft technique, as described by Lord Smith. A disc of the seromuscular layer of the jejunal loop is excised and the mucosa is fixed around a tube, which is then passed through the major duct system of the liver and out of the liver capsule firmly pulling the Roux loop of jejunum into the *porta hepatis.* Mucosal apposition is achieved between the duct system and the jejunum by this technique; thus obviating the need for direct suturing. The tube is removed nine months after surgery. Over the past three years the patient has remained well.

Case 13

A 69-year-old man was admitted as an emergency following an acute attack of upper abdominal colic radiating through to his back. This persisted for 6 hours and was associated with vomiting. The patient had previously experienced several similar attacks of pain which tended to develop in the evening after a heavy meal. There was no history of jaundice but the patient was intolerant of fatty food.

He was tender in the right hypochondrium, Murphy's sign was positive and he was pyrexial with a temperature of 38.2°C.

An ultrasound examination of the gallbladder showed a markedly thickened wall and a solitary stone within it. At laparotomy, the gallbladder was found to be markedly thickened with a mass in the fundus; this had not obviously extended beyond the confines of the serosa of the gallbladder. A cholecystectomy was then performed and operative cholangiography revealed a normal common bile duct with no evidence of choledocholithiasis.

Histological examination of the gallbladder showed a grossly thickened wall which was infiltrated by a poorly differentiated papillary adenocarcinoma. Much of the tumour was necrotic and had spread through the full thickness of the wall to form nodules. One lymph node on the resected specimen contained tumour. The gallbladder elsewhere showed a severe dysplasia amounting to carcinoma *in situ*.

Questions

What course of action should be taken?
What is the prognosis of this condition?

Discussion

Carcinoma of the gallbladder is present in approximately 0.5% of patients undergoing cholecystectomy. It rarely occurs under the age of 60 years and increases thereafter with increasing age. Ninety per cent of patients with carcinoma of the gallbladder also suffer from gallstones. It is probable that the inflammation and infection associated with the stone predispose to malignant change. The mode of spread is chiefly by lymphatics along the cystic duct and thence to the common bile duct. Direct invasion into the liver is a common problem and direct tumour extension often blocks the common bile duct or common hepatic duct producing painless obstructive jaundice.

Following cholecystectomy, the above patient made a good recovery and no further treatment was given. However, 13 months following cholecystectomy, the patient developed jaundice and a second laparotomy revealed multiple hepatic metastases and a huge mass in the *porta hepatis* occluding the common bile duct.

It is debatable whether or not the treatment given to this patient was adequate. Most gallbladder cancers are diagnosed late and inadvertently, as was the case here, for lymph node metastases were present at the time of laparotomy. The crucial prognostic factor is whether or not the tumour has spread through the full thickness of the gallbladder wall to involve the serosa. If confined to the mucosa and submucosa, the 5-year survival rate has been quoted as 63%, and the 10-year survival rate 45%. Conversely, when full thickness involvement of the gallbladder exists, the 5-year survival rate is virtually zero. It has been argued that, in addition to cholecystectomy, wedge resection of approximately 5 cm of normal liver tissue and dissection of the regional lymph nodes should be performed. Where the tumour is advanced and occludes the common bile duct palliative intubation is indicated and, following relief of jaundice, life may be prolonged by up to one year. Radiotherapy and chemotherapy have been used but the response is poor.

The only hope of long-term survival appears to be with early diagnosis. The condition is, however, uncommon and it might be difficult to justify cholecystectomy, even in patients with asymptomatic gallstones, on the grounds of cancer risk alone. Recently there has been a call for conservativism in the treatment of asymptomatic gallstones, but the authors would not endorse this. The mortality for elective cholecystectomy for uncomplicated gallstones is 0.2%, whereas that for obstructive jaundice produced by gallstones is 10% and for gallstone pancreatitis likewise. In the author's view, all patients with gallstones should have a cholecystectomy unless associated medical conditions preclude this. Right hepatic lobectomy has no role in the treatment of gallbladder cancer as the gallbladder lies in the anatomical plane between the right and left lobes of the liver, and both of these lobes are equally likely to become involved with tumour.

On diagnosis of recurrent disease and obstructive jaundice, the only treatment that can be offered is palliative intubation of the duct and relief of jaundice. However, the introduction of a prosthesis may be performed endoscopically, percutaneously and transhepatically and at open operation. The former is probably the best performed at ERCP after endoscopic dilatation of the stricture.

Case 14

A 64-year-old man presented with a 3-week history of anorexia, nausea and the development of jaundice and pruritis. There was no history of weight loss, vomiting or abdominal pain. Examination revealed marked jaundice, but no hepatomegaly and the gallbladder was palpable. His bilirubin concentration was 858 μmol/l, alanine aminotransferase 119 U/l, gamma glutamyl transpeptidase 516 U/l and alkaline phosphatase 1227 U/l. An ultrasound scan showed a dilated bile duct system with gross distension of the gallbladder; no gall stones or liver metastases were present. Chest X-ray showed no abnormality. ERCP revealed a 2.5 cm stenotic lesion in the common bile duct about 5 cm proximal to the ampulla of Vater. The edges of the stricture showed marked shouldering. A percutaneous transhepatic cholangiogram showed dilated intrahepatic biliary radicles with an obstruction just below the junction of the hepatic and cystic ducts.

Questions

What is the diagnosis?
How should the patient be treated?

Discussion

The features present are those of a malignant stricture of the upper common bile duct, most likely due to a cholangiocarcinoma, possibly due to a carcinoma of the pancreas. Expeditious laparotomy is indicated. At operation, a discrete carcinoma of the common bile duct was found, about 2 cm in transverse diameter with its proximal extent lying just below the site of entry of the cystic duct. There was no evidence of lymph node or blood borne metastases. The tumour was mobilised and was found not to invade the portal vein. The common hepatic duct was divided close to its origin and a Whipple's procedure (pancreatico-duodenectomy) was performed.

Malignant tumours of the extra hepatic biliary tree are

uncommon. Being equally distributed between the sexes, they usually occur in the elderly. These tumours are more commonly encountered in the Far East where chronic infestation or suppuration in the biliary tree is more frequent. Although reported to be slow to metastasise, they may be highly lethal.

Where possible, cholangiocarcinomas should be resected and bile drainage re-established by choledocho-jejunostomy using a Roux loop of jejunum. Where the lower extent of the tumour reaches the intrapancreatic portion of the common bile duct, the head of the pancreas and the duodenal loop should be resected. When there is extension into the right and left hepatic ducts, it may be possible to perform individual anastomoses between each of these ducts and the Roux loop. When the tumour occludes both ducts and extends into the liver substance, biliary drainage may be achieved by: (i) Longmire's operation; (ii) anastomosis between an intrahepatic biliary radicle and the gallbladder or (iii) decompression by means of a stent introduced through the tumour substance. In Longmire's operation, the left lobe of the liver is partially resected and a loop of jejunum is anastomosed to the raw surface; this facilitates drainage through one of the large, open, intrahepatic ducts. Anastomosis between an intrahepatic biliary radicle and the gallbladder may be achieved by (i) mobilising the gallbladder from its bed and (ii) dissecting into the liver substance to identify a large intrahepatic bile duct. This can then be anastomosed to the gallbladder inserting a drain to maintain the patency of the anastomosis. Biliary stents may be placed through the stricture either at open operation, percutaneously after dilatation of the stricture or at ERCP again following retrograde dilatation of the malignant stricture.

Radiotherapy has been applied intraoperatively and by ^{192}Ir placed in a stent. Where the disease extends within or is confined to the liver, liver transplantation has been used.

The long-term progress is poor, but improves the lower down the common bile duct the tumour arises. Few patients survive in the long-term when the tumour is situated proximal to the origin of the common bile duct. Those arising in the middle third of the common bile duct have been reported as having a 12% 5-year survival rate and those in the lower third 28%.

Case 15

A 16-year-old girl was admitted to the Accident and Emergency Department having fallen from the pillion seat of a motorbike. She was ultimately thrown into the base of a lamp post, the point of impact being across the upper abdomen. There was bruising across the lower rib cage on the right and tenderness in the right hypochondrium and epigastrium. Chest X-ray showed fractures of the ninth to eleventh ribs on the right; an abdominal X-ray showed no abnormality. At the time of admission there was no sign of shock, but hypotension and tachycardia developed within 1 hour, the pulse rate reaching 100 beats/min and the blood pressure falling from 110/65 mmHg to 90/60 mmHg. By this time, the abdominal tenderness and abdominal girth had both increased.

A needle was inserted into the peritoneal cavity in the right upper quadrant and fresh blood was withdrawn.

Questions

What immediate resuscitative measures are necessary?
What is the surgical approach to this clinical problem?

Discussion

The presence of free intraperitoneal blood in a shocked patient indicates serious visceral damage. The bruising in the right hypochondrium and the fractured ribs are suggestive of liver damage. At the earliest suspicion of such major pathology, blood should be despatched for cross-matching together with a full blood count. Six units of blood should be requested initially; then when the extent of the damage has been established, a request for further blood should be made promptly if major liver damage has occurred. A central venous pressure line is also indicated at an early stage and provides a useful adjunct in the detection of major haemorrhage.

On aspirating blood from the peritoneal cavity urgent laparotomy is indicated. An upper right paramedian incision is appropriate; this can then be extended into a right thoracotomy if necessary. Alternatively, an upper midline incision allows extension into the thoracic cavity by a sternal split if resection is indicated. The right lobe of the liver contained a stellate fracture of the liver pulp with a central 'blow out'. The central defect measured about 8 cm in diameter containing a mass of blood clot. The stellate ramifications breached the capsule at several sites. The left lobe of the liver was intact. Under these circumstances, acute haemorrhage may be temporarily arrested by applying a vascular clamp to those structures in the free border of the lesser omentum which lead to the *porta hepatis* (Pringle's manoeuvre).

In the presence of such extensive destruction of the architecture of the liver, resection of the right lobe is indicated, thus providing the only possibility of permanently arresting haemorrhage. If good facilities and the surgical expertise for liver resection do not exist, then the breach in the liver substance should be packed with large swabs and the patient expeditiously transferred to a major centre.

After removing the gall bladder, the right hepatic duct, artery and right portal vein are ligated and divided, whereupon a plane of demarcation develops between the right and left surgical lobes of the liver. The liver is then resected along this plane using a finger fracture technique and the right hypochondrium is well drained. Following this procedure this patient made an uneventful recovery.

Case 16

A 19-year-old man was admitted after falling from a ladder onto his left side. Since then he had suffered sharp pain in the lower left chest which was exacerbated by deep breathing. He had also become increasingly weak with vague upper abdominal discomfort and pain in the left shoulder.

On examination, he was very pale with a blood pressure of

90/60 mmHg and a weak and thready pulse of 140 min. There was bruising over the left lower ribs and diminished air entry at the left lung base was found. The abdomen was slightly swollen with epigastric and left upper quadrant tenderness and guarding.

Investigations: normal blood chemistry, haemoglobin 8 g/dl with normal indices. Chest X-ray showed fractures of the left eighth and ninth ribs, with an elevated left hemidiaphragm and a small pleural effusion. Abdominal X-ray suggested the presence of intraperitoneal fluid with a typical ground glass appearance.

Questions

What is your diagnosis and how could you confirm it?
How would you manage this patient and what complications might ensue as a result of the treatment?

Discussion

This patient has hypovolaemic shock resulting from sudden loss of blood from the circulation. The position of the injury and the clinical signs all point to a ruptured spleen. Intraperitoneal bleeding can be recognised by intraperitoneal tap with a needle or, more accurately, by peritoneal lavage. This technique is especially useful when a patient is unconscious. Peritoneal lavage is performed after preliminary catheterization of the bladder. A catheter is placed through a small subumbilical stab wound in the abdominal cavity and saline introduced. After withdrawal, the colour of the saline should be viewed. Frank blood and the presence of darkly stained returned saline both indicate significant intra-abdominal bleeding. This patient was initially treated by inserting a wide bore intravenous catheter, and plasma or substitutes (e.g. Haemacel) can be given while waiting for cross-matched blood. If the clinical situation deteriorates rapidly then O negative blood can be used. Pain relief was achieved using parenteral opiates and a urinary catheter was inserted bearing in mind the possibility of renal trauma. A naso-gastric tube was also introduced. Surgery for intraabdominal trauma is usually carried out through a midline incision so that injuries to other abdominal organs can be excluded and treated. During surgery, the abdomen is carefully examined, and any obvious bleeding stopped. If a ruptured spleen is found, the spleen is mobilised and brought into the abdominal wound. If the spleen is severely traumatised, an immediate splenectomy with careful preservation of the pancreatic tail should be performed. If only a small tear is found splenorrhaphy may be indicated although, as yet, this operation is rarely used by surgeons. This procedure may be carried out by using topical haemostatic agents or by using deep sutures.

Portions of the spleen can be transplanted to omental pockets in an attempt to retain some splenic function. At the end of the operation a suction drain is placed into the left upper quadrant. It is essential to perform a full laparotomy as other injuries such as a torn liver or a ruptured duodenum or pancreas can easily be missed. Often retroperitoneal haematomas are found and these should be explored to rule out significant damage to retroperitoneal organs.

The complications of splenectomy encountered in the early postoperative phase are those of respiratory problems and haemorrhage. Atelectasis, especially at the left lung base, is common and can be prevented by adequate physiotherapy and the use of antibiotics.

Postsplenectomy changes in the blood count are invariable and consist of a rise in the white cell count and, more significantly, a rise in platelets. Occasionally, the platelet rise can be so severe as to necessitate treatment to prevent thrombosis. Damage to the pancreas or stomach at operation may produce a postoperative fistula and in rare circumstances a subphrenic abscess.

The major late complication after splenectomy is that of postsplenectomy sepsis. The spleen has a major role in both humoral and cell mediated immunity. It produces opsonins (e.g. tuftsin and properdin) which are important in the phagocytosis of encapsulated bacteria (e.g. pneumococcus). When postsplenectomy sepsis occurs there is a very high mortality rate, particularly in young patients. Postsplenectomy sepsis may be prevented by the use of vaccines such as Pneumovac and by long-term use of low-dose penicillin. Indeed, the historical concept of the spleen as a superfluous organ is obviously false when one considers the problems of postsplenectomy sepsis.

There are also reports that patients having undergone splenectomy are more at risk of developing ischaemic heart disease in later years.

Case 17

A 47-year-old female when admitted to hospital for a minor gynaecological procedure, was found to have a discrete large mass in the right hypochondrium. She had hitherto been totally asymptomatic with regard to the mass. An ultrasound scan showed a grossly enlarged right lobe of the liver with a central large mass and surrounding smaller swellings within the liver substance. There was no past history of hepatitis nor of alcohol abuse, the patient had always lived in the U.K. Computerised tomography confirmed the presence of a mass in the right lobe of the liver with a possible extension along the vessels in the *porta hepatis* and posterior to the pancreas. Biochemical tests of liver function were normal, except a raised alkaline phosphatase 343 U/l. The chest X-ray was normal.

Questions

What further investigations are appropriate?
What treatment is indicated?

Discussion

As the mass was both palpable and easily imaged by ultrasound, an ultrasound guided needle biopsy of the hepatic mass was performed after excluding a coagulation abnormality. This showed the presence of either a small cell tumour, possibly of the APUD variety, or alternatively a hepatocellular carcinoma. Urine was despatched for 5-HIAA and serum for a 'gut hormone profile' and for α-fetoprotein estimation. Upper gastrointestinal endoscopy revealed the presence of a superficial duodenal ulcer. The urine was negative for 5-HIAA but the serum α-fetoprotein level was 20 000 ng/ml.

A laparotomy was performed through a right paramedian incision. A tumour occupied most of the right liver lobe which was grossly enlarged by its presence. The left lobe of the liver appeared disease free. The under surface of the diaphragm and the posterior aspect of the anterior abdominal wall were invaded by tumour over the surface of which coursed some large blood vessels. Tumour extended from the *porta hepatis* along the major vessels and bile duct and posterior to the neck of the pancreas. Resection of the right lobe of the liver was not possible. A wedge biopsy of the tumour was taken for further histological examination and for oestrogen receptor assay. One week after the initial α-fetoprotein estimation, the level had doubled to 40 000 ng/ml. The wedge biopsy confirmed the diagnosis of hepatocellular carcinoma.

Question

What further treatment was available?

Discussion

Here we are confronted with a very aggressive tumour with a doubling time of approximately one week. No known predisposing factors to hepatocellular carcinoma such as alcohol abuse, hepatitis B surface antigen positive status or dwelling in an area of high incidence were present.

All that can be offered to patients with such advanced hepatocellular carcinoma is chemotherapy or possibly embolisation of the hepatic artery. Chemotherapy has not yielded very encouraging results, although currently adriamycin is widely used. Chemotherapeutic agents have been introduced directly into the liver following selective catheterisation of the hepatic artery, but the results of this form of therapy have also been disappointing. Hepatic artery occlusion by embolisation or direct surgical ligation has been advocated for patients unsuitable for surgical resection; it is, however, contraindicated in the presence of portal vein involvement by tumour. Revascularisation from the hepatic capsular vessels rapidly occurs following embolisation and convincing evidence of prolongation of life has not been demonstrated. Recently, oestrogen receptors have been found in some hepatocellular carcinomas, thus tamoxifen is now frequently used together with, or instead of, chemotherapeutic agents. There is, as yet, no convincing evidence of its value.

Unless the disease is confined to one lobe of the liver and is thus resectable, the prognosis is very poor, most unresectable patients living less than 1 year.

Case 18

A 42-year-old man was admitted as an emergency following a haematemesis. He had vomited a large amount of blood on arriving home from a public house and this had led to a period of vertigo and ataxia. For several days prior to this episode, he had passed melaena stools. The patient began drinking beer to excess at the age of eighteen years; he changed to champagne and brandy, but when his financial resources prohibited this, he again began drinking beer. At the time of presentation he was drinking approximately 12 pints of beer each night.

Examination revealed a pale man with a distended abdomen but no masses were present. There were no clinical manifestations of liver disease other than spider naevi. Soon after admission he had a further haematemesis and passed fresh blood per rectum. He became shocked but responded to blood transfusion.

Gastroduodenoscopy revealed large oesophageal varices and a duodenal ulcer, the latter having a visible vessel in the base.

The patient was treated with cimetidine (400 mg b.d.) and a conventional antacid (magnesium trisilicate). His bleeding stopped, but before further investigations could be performed the patient discharged himself from hospital and failed to attend for follow-up. Liver biochemistry showed raised alanine aminotransferase (56 U/l), gamma glutamyl transpeptidase (137 U/l) and alkaline phosphatase (167 U/l).

Six months later he was again admitted as an emergency with a haematemesis following a bout of heavy drinking. His haemoglobin concentration was 7.6 g/dl and liver function tests were essentially unchanged, with the exception of bilirubin concentration which was now marginally elevated at 25 μmol/l.

Questions

How should his gastrointestinal tract bleeding be managed? What is the long-term management of the underlying condition?

Discussion

The first priority in medical management is to correct the state of shock. Intravenous fluids are administered and, initially, six units of blood should be cross-matched. As soon as possible gastroduodenoscopy should be performed. On the initial admission, although oesophageal varices were present, this patient was bleeding from a peptic ulcer. In approximately 35% of patients with oesophageal varices the bleeding results from causes other than the oesophageal varices themselves, most commonly a peptic ulcer. On the second admission, the oesophageal varices were bleeding from a point 2 cm from the gastro-oesophageal junction.

It is common practice to infuse vasopressin (pitressin) which lowers portal venous pressure by constricting the vessels in the splanchnic arteriolar bed. This is usually given as an intravenous infusion of 20 units in 200 ml of 5% dextrose over a ten-minute period; alternatively, a slow infusion of 0.4 units/min may be given over two hours. Patients with a history of ischaemic heart disease should not be given vasopressin as there is a risk of inducing a myocardial infarction due to vasoconstriction. Propranolol has recently been advocated both for use in the acute variceal bleed and as a prophylaxis against further bleeding.

If bleeding continues, balloon tamponade provides an effective short-term method of controlling haemorrhage. The four-lumen Minnesota tube is most commonly used, and has two balloons. The gastric balloon is inflated to a volume of 300 ml and tension is applied by impacting this balloon in the gastric fundus. The oesophageal balloon is then inflated to a pressure of 40 mm Hg, using a sphygmomanometer, thus arresting haemorrhage by direct variceal compression. The oesophageal balloon should be deflated after 18 hours and if haemorrhage has been arrested the Minnesota tube is removed. These balloons, when carefully used, are effective in arresting haemorrhage in over 90% of cases; however, there is a 60% incidence of early rebleeding.

Once the haemorrhage has abated, injection sclerotherapy may be used. Using either a flexible or rigid endoscope, the varices are directly injected with up to 25 ml of ethanolamine oleate given in divided 2–3 ml alliquots. Using this technique bleeding is controlled, in the short-term, in approximately 90% of cases. Repeated sclerosis is, however, essential on a 2–3 weekly basis until the varices have been completely sclerosed. An alternative method to sclerosis is transection of the oesophagus using a stapling gun. Through an anterior gastrotomy the oesophagus is stapled by passing the EEA circular stapling device into the lower oesophagus, which is stapled 1–2 cm above the oesophago-gastric junction.

Portasystemic shunts are now used much less frequently than hitherto was the case, particularly in the alcoholic cirrhotic with portal hypertension. The mortality in the acute bleeding situation is at least 50%, although, when performed electively the mortality is much lower. A high proportion of cirrhotic patients develop hepatic encephalopathy and liver failure after porta-caval anastomosis. Warren advocates the use of a distal spleno-renal anastomosis, which is complicated by a much lower incidence of hepatic encephalopathy; whether overall survival is improved has not firmly been established.

Stopping the patient drinking is imperative to long-term survival, but is rarely achieved. Although this patient's disease is currently in the Child's B category, his continued drinking and failure to comply with medical and psychiatric treatment mean that it is unlikely that he will survive for more than 1 or 2 years.

Case 19

A 46-year-old man presented with increasing abdominal distension. Three years earlier he had been diagnosed as suffering from chronic alcoholic liver disease. Since then he had stopped taking alcohol completely and, although his liver showed no signs of clinical deterioration, his ascites continued to recur. He had undergone multiple paracenteses and had failed to respond to medical management. During the same period he had become increasingly weak and had lost over 2 stones in weight.

On examination, he was a thin wasted man with several spider naevi on the face. There was no evidence of jaundice or other signs of liver failure. Gross distension of the abdomen was present, but there was no evidence of dilated peri-umbilical veins. Rectal examination was unremarkable and, in particular, there was no evidence of a shelf of tumour in the pouch of Douglas. Ankle swelling was also present.

Investigations

Haemoglobin 10.2 g/dl. White cell count 9.3 x 10⁹/l. Electrolytes normal. Urea 16.5 mmol/l. Creatinine 250 mmol/l, bilirubin 19 μmol/l, ALT 56 U/l, alkaline phosphatase 250 U/l. Total protein 75 g/l, albumin 31 g/l, prothrombin time ratio 1.3:1. Chest X-ray was normal. Abdominal X-ray confirmed the presence of intraperitoneal fluid.

Questions

What is the differential diagnosis in this patient?
How should this patient's ascites be best managed?

Discussion

The presence of fluid or ascites within the peritoneal cavity may be related to a variety of disease processes. Chronic liver disease such as cirrhosis related to alcoholism, primary biliary cirrhosis and chronic active hepatitis are commonly associated with ascites. In addition, the Budd-Chiari syndrome gives marked ascites. Malignancy within the peritoneal cavity from primaries such as ovary, bowel, breast and lung frequently causes marked ascites. Less commonly, ascites is related to pancreatic causes such as a pseudocyst or traumatic rupture of the duct. Chylous ascites may occur following damage to the cisterna chyli. In tropical areas, tuberculous ascites is common.

The presence of ascites is usually apparent on clinical examination. When relatively small amounts of fluid are present, shifting dullness may be elicited. If large amounts of fluid are free within the peritoneal cavity then a fluid thrill should be easily felt.

Symptoms and signs of liver failure and metastatic carcinoma must be sought for. In addition, rectal examination and vaginal examination are imperative to exclude the presence of pelvic carcinomatosis. Widespread wasting of muscles is often associated with hypoalbuminaemia in the presence of ascites.

The mainstay of management of ascites is firstly to determine the cause of the fluid accumulation. In the presence of suspected ascites, a needle can be inserted into the peritoneal cavity and fluid aspirated. This fluid should be examined carefully by cytology for the presence of malignant cells, by microbiology for bacteria and biochemically for the presence of amylase and the protein level. Where liver disease is suspected, varices should be excluded by means of gastroscopy or barium meal. A liver and spleen isotope scan may also be beneficial. Primary liver disease should be investigated by means of ultrasonography and liver biopsy. Extreme care must be taken in performing liver biopsy in patients with marked ascites since there is a high incidence of haemorrhagic complications. In the presence of marked ascites, it is probably safer to perform liver biopsy under laparoscopic control. The presence of widespread carcinomatosis must be carefully excluded by means of chest X-ray and bone scan. In this patient, the cause of ascites was the presence of long-standing liver damage. The liver damage in cirrhosis results in portal hypertension; this causes a transudate containing low levels of protein into the peritoneal cavity. Cardiac failure, the Budd-Chiari syndrome and hypo-albuminaemia may also cause a transudate. An exudate containing high levels of protein is caused by the presence of inflammation within the peritoneal cavity and widespread carcinomatosis, where damaged capillaries allow the escape of proteins. An exudate is associated with a protein level of greater than 30 g/l whereas transudates have a protein level of less than this. Recently the level of lactic dehydrogenase has been measured in the ascitic fluid. When this is greater than that of the serum, ascites almost certainly results from carcinomatosis. When the level is lower, ascites probably results from cirrhosis and liver damage.

The primary treatment in these patients involves managing the liver problem itself and treating liver failure. Diuretics are given to combat ascites, the most effective of these being spironolactone, which reverses the secondary hyper-aldosteronism common in these patients. Other diuretics such as frusemide and amiloride may also be given. When ascites is very marked, paracentesis can be performed; however, this procedure may be dangerous as rapid removal of fluid may cause shock with hypovolaemia and hypoproteinaemia. Most patients with ascites due to cirrhosis respond to a combination of paracentesis and diuretic therapy. A small group of patients however, require, further management.

Ascites due to carcinomatosis should be treated by systemic therapy. In particular, ovarian carcinoma should be treated by chemotherapy and breast carcinoma by chemotherapy or endocrine manipulation. Successful treatment of these primary carcinomas will often cause spontaneous regression of ascites. A pancreatic cause for ascites should be suspected by the presence of a high amylase level within the peritoneal fluid and damage to the pancreatic duct must be confirmed on ERCP investigation. Tuberculous and other infective causes of ascites should be treated with the appropriate antibiotics.

Resistant ascites related to liver failure or disseminated malignancy has recently been treated by the placement of a peritoneovenous shunt. Two shunts have been described namely the Leveen shunt and the Denver shunt and these shunts carry ascitic fluid from the peritoneal cavity to the jugular vein. Although both shunts have their advantages and disadvantages, their effectiveness appears to be similar. The shunt itself can be inserted either under local or general anaesthetic. A small hole is made in the peritoneum and a plastic tube bearing multiple holes is inserted. The tube is then tunnelled over the ribcage and the other end inserted into the external jugular vein. A valve or pumping chamber is present halfway along the tube and should be positioned over a rib, since this allows the patient to pump the tube himself to prevent obstruction. Several contra-indications to the placement of a peritoneovenous shunt have been described and these are (i) infection within the peritoneal cavity, (ii) terminal disease, (iii) the presence of blood-stained ascites (iv) a very high protein level in the ascitic fluid of greater than 50 g/l, (v) loculated ascites and (vi) jaundice. Several complications relate to the placement of these shunts. Many patients develop a fever of unknown origin. Disseminated intravascular coagulation occasionally occurs although its likelihood can be reduced by removing all ascitic fluid when the shunt is initially inserted. Shunt occlusion is common and is related to the deposition of fibrin and omentum plugging the intraperitoneal part of the tube. When blockage occurs, ascitic fluid will rapidly build up and can be detected by ultrasonography. In such patients, the tube should be removed and replaced. The presence of a pumping chamber halfway along the tube has helped to reduce this complication.

Dissemination of malignant cells through the shunt in the presence of widespread carcinomatosis within the periotoneal cavity does not appear to cause a clinical deterioration. These cells appear to be trapped in the pulmonary capillaries and do not lead to overt metastases in the rest of the body.

In selected patients with resistant ascites, peritoneovenous shunts have an important role. They do not specifically prolong life but improve the quality of life.

Case 20

A 49-year-old man presented with a 1-year history of severe epigastric pain, with an initial onset 1–2 hours after meals and being alleviated by antacids and later H_2-receptor antagonists. The pain subsequently became progressively severe and almost continuous. Four years previously, the patient had undergone truncal vagotomy and pyloroplasty for a chronic duodenal ulcer. As the severity of the pain had increased, the patient also developed vomiting and diarrhoea and had experienced one episode of upper gastrointestinal tract bleeding.

Upper gastrointestinal tract endoscopy showed an aggressive peptic ulcer diathesis with multiple ulcers situated in the first and second parts of the duodenum.

Questions

What is the likely diagnosis?
How should the patient further be investigated?
What treatment is indicated for this condition?

Discussion

The most common cause of recurrent peptic ulceration after a previous vagotomy is incomplete division of the vagus nerve. If only 10% of the total vagal innervation to the stomach is left intact, the whole mucosal syncitium can become re-innervated. However, in this case the aggressive nature of the ulcer diathesis and the development of diarrhoea makes the diagnosis of Zollinger-Ellison syndrome much more likely than recurrent peptic ulceration due to incomplete vagotomy. Serum gastrin estimation was performed under fasting conditions and found to be 740 pg/ml which is markedly above the upper limit of normal (200 pg/ml) and suggests the diagnosis of the Zollinger–Ellison syndrome. This may be confirmed by the infusion of either calcium or secretin. After intravenous administration of calcium (15 mg/kg/3-hourly) a rise in the gastrin level of 300 pg/ml is diagnostic and after administering secretin as a bolus (2 IU/

kg intravenously) a rise of 100 pg/ml is also diagnostic. Serum calcium estimation should be carried out and, if elevated, would suggest the presence of a parathyroid adenoma in addition to a gastrinoma as part of a multiple endocrine adenopathy (MEA). A test of gastric secretory function should also be performed. It is our practice to carry out a combined insulin and pentagastrin test. After an overnight fast the stomach is intubated and aspirated. Thereafter basal secretions are collected for 30 minutes and a bolus dose of insulin 0.2 IU/kg is given intravenously. After a 90-minute period pentagastrin (6µg/kg, subcutaneously) is given and secretions are collected for a further hour. A basal acid output of 9 mmol/hour is highly suggestive of the Zollinger–Ellison syndrome. Also a high basal to maximal acid output ratio is suggestive of the Zollinger–Ellison syndrome since it indicates that the parietal cells are already near to maximal stimulation by endogenous gastrin. Either an ultrasound scan or CT scan of the upper abdomen should be performed to identify a pancreatic tumour. Selective venous sampling following catheterisation of the splenic vein may be helpful in anatomically localising the presence of a gastrinoma. Selective angiography may also be effective in demonstrating the presence of a tumour circulation within the pancreas.

Having established the diagnosis, the patient should initially be treated by an H_2-receptor antagonist in double the recommended dosage; this treatment should be continued prior to surgery.

Sixty per cent of these tumours undergo malignant change, and this is the major argument in favour of surgical treatment since the earlier the tumour is detected the better the chance of cure.

At operation, the disease should be staged, the pancreas and adjacent lymph nodes being carefully examined along the liver. Where a single tumour is identified in the body or tail of the gland distal pancreatectomy is indicated. Tumours in the head of the pancreas require excision by Whipple's operation. Total pancreatectomy is seldom required and, on occasions, local excision of an adenoma may be possible.

As an adjunct to tumour excision, if the patient has not previously undergone vagotomy, highly selective vagotomy should be performed. Where the tumour is quite clearly malignant with extra-pancreatic spread, as much of the tumour mass as possible should be removed and the patient may then be treated by streptozocin. The potent antisecretory drug omeprazole may have a role in the management of these cases.

The original surgical treatment used for this condition was total gastrectomy, which cured the ulcer and remained standard therapy for some 20 years. It still has a role, either when the tumour has metastasised widely and is producing intractable ulceration, or when the primary neoplasm cannot be identified.

Case 21

A 36-year-old woman was admitted with a 24-hour history of pain in the right hypochondrium, spreading across the upper abdomen and radiating into the back. At the time of admission to hospital there was upper abdominal tenderness, but no other abnormality. The patient had a history of several attacks of epigastric and subcostal pain and some intolerance to fatty food. Over the next two hours, the upper abdominal tenderness markedly increased, bowel sounds became absent and a tachycardia developed with a fall in blood pressure from 130/80 to 110/75 mmHg. Full blood count on admission was normal, as were chest and plain abdominal X-rays; however, the serum amylase was elevated to 600 U/l.

Questions

What is the differential diagnosis?
What further investigations should be performed?
What treatment should be carried out for this patient?

Discussion

The most likely diagnosis is acute pancreatitis but, at this stage, perforated peptic ulcer and acute cholecystitis or biliary colic should still be considered.

Though elevated, the serum amylase is not yet high enough to be diagnostic of acute pancreatitis. Paradoxically, not all patients with acute pancreatitis have a serum amylase estimation in excess of 1000 U/l which is the accepted level above which the diagnosis of acute pancreatitis can quite definitely be made. Similarly, there is no direct correlation between the level of serum amylase and the severity of pancreatitis. Those with a severe form of necrotising haemorrhagic pancreatitis often destroy their pancreas so rapidly as not to release sufficient amylase into the blood stream, thereby failing to reach the above diagnostic threshold. In addition, the timing of the blood sample may be crucial as the serum level of amylase may rise and fall quickly and the sample may be taken as the amylase is either rising or falling. In this patient, a repeat amylase estimation six hours later revealed a concentration of 2634 U/l, confirming the diagnosis of acute pancreatitis. Chest and plain abdominal X-ray must always be performed. During the early stages of the disorder the former is most likely to be normal, the latter may show a dilated 'sentinel loop' of small intestine in the periumbilical region. An ultrasound scan of the gallbladder, biliary tract and pancreas should be performed to exclude the presence of cholelithiasis or pancreatic enlargement. In this patient multiple small stones were seen within the gallbladder.

No specific form of drug therapy has been shown to beneficially to influence the course of an attack of acute pancreatitis. Treatment is chiefly supportive and aimed at preventing or treating complications; most patients recover spontaneously regardless of specific therapy. Those with severe manifestations of their disease should be managed in an intensive care unit.

The prognosis varies widely between the two extremes of the disease, thus making early diagnosis of the severe case important. In such patients mortality increases: (i) over the age of 55 years; (ii) with pre-existing diabetes; (iii) with a low arterial pO_2, (iv) with low calcium and albumin levels and (v) with respiratory and renal insufficiency. Elevated blood urea, creatinine and bilirubin levels with concomitant low levels of parathormone and the presence of methaemalbumin also indicate severe disease.

Patients with the mild disease require intravenous fluid replacement with nasogastric aspiration and analgesics such as pethidine or morphine and Buscopan. The patient with the severe disease may, in addition, require plasma, calcium and oxygen; on occasions, positive pressure ventilation is required together with treatment of incipient or established renal failure.

Early cholecystectomy and operative cholangiography should be favoured in established gallstone pancreatitis. When this is delayed the incidence of choledocholithiasis at operation is no greater than that in patients undergoing a cholecystectomy without a history of pancreatitis; however, when surgery is performed within 48 hours of the onset of the attack, stones are present in the lower common bile duct in 75% of cases.

The exact optimal time for surgery remains controversial. Protagonists of early surgery emphasize the established observation that recurrent attacks are likely to occur unless the biliary tract disease has been eradicated. In a recent report, 92% of patients presenting with recurrent bile duct stones after cholecystectomy for gallstone pancreatitis had further attacks of pancreatitis.

In those patients operated upon six to eight weeks after an attack 25% will have a further attack of pancreatitis or acute cholecystitis during this time. Most surgeons would now operate when the pancreatitis has clinically resolved during the first hospital admission (usually within one to two weeks). Operation within 48 hours of admission has also been recommended and shown to be associated with a high incidence of common bile duct stones at operation and a low mortality.

Early endoscopic papillotomy and removal of stones has recently been advocated, further results of this technique are awaited.

Case 22

A 65-year-old man presented with a 48-hour history of increasing epigastric pain which was continuous, unrelated to food and radiated through to the back. There was no past history of similar pain. On close questioning, he admitted to a high alcohol consumption for at least six years prior to admission.

On examination, he appeared unwell and was pale, sweaty and cyanosed. The blood pressure was 80/50 mmHg, the pulse 120/min and thready. Examination of the abdomen revealed diffuse tenderness, most marked in the epigastrium. There were no signs of alcoholic liver disease and no evidence of jaundice. Breath sounds were reduced over the left lower lobe.

Investigations

Sodium 130 mmol/l. Potassium 4.6 mmol/l. Urea 25 mmol/l. Creatinine 310 μmol/l. Haemoglobin 10.6 g/dl. White count 17.8×10^9/l. Glucose 16.5 mmol/l. Blood gases, PO_2 7.3 kPa. PCO_2 4.8 kPa. Chest X-ray revealed a small effusion at the left base. Abdominal X-ray showed evidence of dilated small bowel but no free gas. The serum amylase concentration was 1120 U/l.

Questions

What is the differential diagnosis?
How may the severity of the disease be assessed?
What treatments are available and what are their effects on the course of the disease?

Discussion

The most likely diagnosis in this patient is acute pancreatitis. However, several other conditions are associated with severe upper abdominal pain, shock and a raised amylase. These include a ruptured abdominal aortic aneurysm (which can be excluded by clinical examination where a pulsatile mass is present in the epigastrium), acute cholecystitis, perforated peptic (ulcer which may be excluded by the absence of free gas on X-ray) and superior mesenteric artery occlusion. If there is any doubt about the diagnosis of pancreatitis, then laparotomy should be performed after initial resuscitation.

The commonest cause of acute pancreatitis in young patients is alcohol abuse and in older patients gallstones. In the United Kingdom gallstones account for approximately 50–60% of cases of pancreatitis, with alcohol accounting for approximately 10–15%. In a small group of patients no identifiable cause can be found. Acute pancreatitis is associated with the release of toxic substances from the pancreas which pass into the peritoneum and into the general circulation and thus result in severe generalised disease. Although the presence of a raised amylase level is probably the most useful indicator of the presence of acute pancreatitis, occasionally the diagnosis is made only at laparotomy or on peritoneal lavage. Having made the diagnosis of acute pancreatitis, the next most important step is to differentiate the clinically severe attack from the mild form of the disease.

Acute haemorrhagic pancreatitis has a mortality rate of approximately 80% in contrast to interstitial or oedematous pancreatitis which generally run a benign course. Several clinical signs point to the presence of severe disease and these include shock, cyanosis, a rigid abdomen and bruising both in the loin (Grey–Turner sign) and periumbilically (Cullen's sign). Clinical evaluation alone, however, has a low predictive value in the determination of severe disease. Thus several indices have been devised objectively to determine the severity of the disease process at an early stage. These indices use clinical and biochemical parameters present within 48 hours of admission. The two most commonly employed indices are those of Ransom and Imrie. Factors indicating severe disease include: hypoxia ($pO_2 \leq 8$ kPa), high blood glucose, rising urea and creatinine levels, falling haematocrit, elevated LDH and ALT levels, high white cell count, low serum calcium, fluid sequestration, metabolic acidosis and the presence of a 'prune juice' coloured fluid aspirate on peritoneal lavage. The presence of methaemalbumen and elevated serum ribonuclease enzyme have also been suggested as parameters of severe damage.

This patient demonstrates many signs of severe disease both from the biochemical estimations and the clinical presentation.

Treatment of patients with acute haemorrhagic pancreatitis is difficult and requires management in an intensive care unit. Intravenous fluids must be given in large quantities; frequently plasma or blood are also needed. A central venous pressure line and urinary catheter are useful in assessing fluid balance and a Swan–Ganz catheter may be of value in severe cases. The blood pressure should be maintained above 120 mmHg to prevent renal failure developing. Pain relief is essential in these patients and pethidine is usually used in preference to morphine as the latter produces more marked and prolonged constriction of the sphincter of Oddi. Gastric dilation and ileus are frequently associated with severe pancreatitis and a nasogastric tube must be used in these patients. Oxygen must be administered in high concentrations to correct the severe hypoxia often found in these patients. Where respiratory problems become manifest assisted ventilation may be needed.

Various drugs have been used in an attempt to reduce the severity of pancreatitis and these include trasylol and glucagon. Several studies have shown, however, that they have little effect. Antibiotics should probably be given to all patients with acute hamorrhagic pancreatitis although their efficacy is not proven. When metabolic abnormalities such as metabolic acidosis, hypocalcaemia and hyperglycaemia occur these should be corrected by the judicious use of bicarbonate calcium and insulin respectively.

Despite the treatments already mentioned there is no doubt that the most important part in the management of these patients is the prevention of shock and hypotension. Dissatisfaction with the results of treatment of haemorrhagic pancreatitis has resulted in several new methods of therapy. Peritoneal lavage has recently been advocated; however, a randomised controlled trial showed that it had no effect on either morbidity or mortality associated with the condition. Exchange transfusion has also been proposed as being of benefit in this disease although its effectiveness is as yet unproven. Likewise phospholipase inhibitors may be of value although they are as yet unproven.

Laparotomy may be performed if there is doubt about the diagnosis. In the necrotising form of the disease the pancreas is seen to be enlarged, black and haemorrhagic and the abdominal cavity is usually filled with a dark-stained fluid ('prune juice'). The peritoneal cavity should be lavaged and drains placed into the lesser sac to allow irrigation and drainage of the peripancreatic area. Some surgeons advocate pancreatectomy, although this operation is accompanied by a very high mortality in these situations. Later in the course of the disease, when there is evidence of extensive tissue necrosis, sepsis and ongoing pancreatic inflammation, then limited resection should be performed. Computerised tomography (CT) is useful in selecting patients who might benefit from these desloughing procedures.

Acute haemorrhagic pancreatitis is associated with several severe and life-threatening complications. Of these, respiratory failure is the most important. Pancreatitis affects the lungs in several ways: (i) by destroying surfactant in the alveoli, (ii) by depositing fibrin in the alveolar walls and (iii) by causing pleural effusions. These result in severe hypoxia and frequently acute respiratory distress syndrome or shock lung develops. These patients are best managed using oxygen therapy, although there has been recent interest in the use of heparin. The ischaemic and necrotic pancreas releases a substance termed 'myocardial depressant factor' into the circulation, and this serves to further complicate the shock of these patients.

Renal failure is common in patients with haemorrhagic pancreatitis and is related to shock, hypovolaemia and toxins released from the pancreas. When it occurs, dialysis may be needed but frequently the renal failure results from irreversible acute cortical necrosis. The maintenance of a near-normal blood pressure and urine output are vital in preventing renal failure. Liver failure with jaundice may also occur, as may disseminated intravascular coagulation and bleeding disorders.

Within the abdomen itself pancreatic inflammation may erode blood vessels thus causing a major haemorrhage; this is frequently the cause of death in these patients. In addition abscesses may occur, especially in the retroperitoneum and these require drainage.

After resolution of acute inflammation, pancreatitis can persist and cause pseudocysts. Most pseudocysts are small and can only be detected using ultrasonography. When large pseudocysts require drainage to prevent bleeding and rupture, this can be performed by cystogastrostomy or cysto-jejunostomy Roux-en-Y. Fistulae from the pancreas, biliary tree, stomach and small bowel may also occur. Pancreatic inflammation may extend into the surrounding tissues causing necrosis of the duodenum and colon and, in severe cases, the entire retroperitoneal space may be destroyed by ongoing inflammation.

The overall mortality in patients with acute haemorrhagic pancreatitis is approximately 70 to 80%. Increasing numbers of poor risk factors, using the severity indices of Ransom and Imrie, are associated with an increasingly poor prognosis.

Case 23

A 46-year-old man presented with a 3-year history of increasing epigastric pain. This pain was situated just above the umbilicus and radiated through to the back. There were no precipitating factors and, in particular, the pain was not related to food. He had also noticed increasingly loose bowel motions and recently had been discovered by his general practitioner to be mildly diabetic. On close questioning he admitted to a moderately large alcohol intake mostly consisting of spirits.

On examination, he was a thin, gaunt man. There was evidence of mild icterus but no signs of liver failure. Examination of the abdomen revealed slight tenderness in the epigastrium with no evidence of hepato-splenomegaly and no masses could be felt.

Investigations

Urea and electrolytes, normal. Bilirubin 65 μmol/l. Alkaline phosphatase 330U/l, ALT 40U/l, Gamma glutamyl transpeptidase 350U/l. Full blood count was normal apart from a slightly elevated MCV of 105 fl. Fasting blood glucose 16 mmol/l with glycosuria noticed on urinalysis. Stool culture was normal and faecal fat excretion was greater than 10 g in 24 hours. Chest X-ray normal. Abdominal X-ray revealed calcification on both sides of the lumbar spine in the region of the L1 vertebra. Gastroscopy was normal, as was an oral cholecystogram.

Questions

Discuss the investigations of this patient and your likely diagnosis.
How may this patient be managed both medically and surgically?

Discussion

The key features to notice in this patient are the long history of alcohol abuse associated with epigastric pain radiating through to the back, mild diabetes, steatorrhoea and jaundice. The presence of calcification in the upper abdomen is almost diagnostic of chronic alcoholic pancreatitis.

It is important in this case to exclude other causes of upper abdominal pain such as peptic ulceration, aortic aneurysm, pancreatic carcinoma, gallstones and gastric carcinoma. Gastroscopy is mandatory and, in this patient, there was no evidence of a peptic ulceration or gastric carcinoma. The liver function tests suggest obstructive jaundice and this was investigated using ultrasonography. This demonstrated dilatation of the intra- and extra-hepatic bile ducts with a blockage at the lower end of the common bile duct. The gallbladder was enlarged but there was no evidence of stones. The liver appeared to be normal. Although ultrasonographic examination of the pancreas was difficult, there was a suggestion of enlargement of the gland in association with several small cysts. CT is often of benefit in assessing pancreatic pathology and, in this case, the pancreas was seen to be enlarged with three or four small cysts identified along the length of the gland. The common bile duct was also dilated. There was no evidence of any mass lesion such as carcinoma of the pancreas.

In those patients where the diagnosis of chronic pancreatitis is less obvious, pancreatic function tests may be of value. These tests include duodenal intubation with a collection of pancreatic fluid after stimulation by secretin and pancreozymin. A recently developed PABA test may also be of value in distinguishing chronic pancreatitis from other causes of upper abdominal pain. Glucose tolerance tests should be performed in all patients with suspected chronic pancreatitis to exclude the possibility of diabetes. Steator-rhoea is often seen in these patients but is frequently a late feature of advanced disease. Faecal fat estimation is of benefit in assessing the degree of fat malabsorption related to pancreatic insufficiency.

The most useful investigative tool at the present time is endoscopic retrograde cholangiopancreatography (ERCP). In this investigation a side viewing endoscope is passed into the duodenum and the ampulla of Vater cannulated. Dye is injected into the biliary tree and the presence or absence of gallstones and blockage to the biliary tree assessed. Dye is then injected into the pancreatic duct to obtain a pancreatogram.

Chronic pancreatitis is associated with varying degrees of duct damage dependent on the severity and extent of the disease. Mild disease results in slight irregularities to side ducts, whereas severe disease is associated with almost complete blockage of the main pancreatic duct, a grossly enlarged pancreatic duct and the presence of several cysts in a 'chain of lakes' appearance. These films can also be assessed for the presence or absence of suspected carcinoma of the pancreas. It is important to realise that carcinoma of the pancreas may superimpose itself upon co-existing chronic pancreatitis and it is therefore vital that this disease be excluded.

In this patient full ERCP examination was impossible because of biliary tract obstruction. There was, however, evidence of ampullary swelling and, when dye was injected into the pancreatic duct this was dilated with gross ductular distortion and dilatation. In situations where the lower biliary tree cannot be cannulated a percutaneous transhepatic cholangiogram should be performed. In this patient, this showed evidence of a smooth narrowing of the lower end of the common bile duct suggestive of blockage by chronic pancreatitis.

Chronic pancreatitis is most commonly resultant upon alcohol abuse, although other causes such as haemachromatosis and drug addiction are recognised. In many cases, however, no single cause can be identified. The pathological findings are those of deposition of protein plugs in the pancreatic ducts resulting in blockage of these ducts. Later these protein plugs become calcified. This leads to intense pain and progressive pancreatic damage with fibrosis. The fibrosis also involves the Islets of Langerhans, which results in diabetes. When fibrosis affects the head of the gland, this can also involve the terminal common bile duct, as in this patient, and result in obstructive jaundice. Narrowing of the ducts results in a build-up of pancreatic secretions and the formation of cysts. Gradually the pancreatic tissue becomes progressively destroyed with loss of remaining pancreatic function. The pain associated with chronic pancreatitis is often severe and may be due to irritation of the coeliac plexus, inflammatory changes causing distortion of the capsule of the gland and blockage of the ducts.

The treatment of patients with chronic pancreatitis is frequently difficult in view of coexistent alcoholism. Medical management should be first employed in all cases and the most important feature of management must be insistence on the complete abstinence from alcohol. Indeed, persistent alcohol intake will result in further pancreatic damage, with a vicious circle often developing with the patient consuming alcohol for short-term relief and inducing further pain. Pain relief must be adequate but may, unless care is exerted, result in drug dependence. The diabetes in these patients is often unstable because of alcohol abuse and may require either oral hypoglycaemic agents or insulin. The lack of pancreatic enzymes results in malabsorption leading to diarrhoea and steatorrhoea. These enzymes can be replaced by several pancreatic supplements including Cotazyme and Pancreozyme; H_2-blockers are also needed to prevent their destruction in the stomach.

The role of surgery in the treatment of these patients remains controversial. This is due, in part, to the fact that these patients are frequently alcoholic and will continue drinking after surgery. Also there is doubt as to whether surgery reduces pain and improves the quality of life. However, the presence of jaundice, as in this patient, is a definite indication for surgery. As the blockage is at the lower end of the common bile duct and the gallbladder is normal, a simple bypass operation such as cholecystjejunostomy can be employed to good effect. If there is evidence of duodenal obstruction resultant on pancreatic inflammation, then a gastroenterostomy should also be performed.

Surgical therapy to the pancreas itself depends upon the distribution of duct abnormalities demonstrated on ERCP. Operative pancreatography is an alternative method of outlining the pancreatic ducts. The multiplicity of procedures recommended for the surgical treatment of pancreatitis indicates the failure of any one operation to satisfy the needs of all patients and emphasises that different operative procedures may be required at varying stages in the disease process. Every patient must be individually assessed, and the extent and nature of the disease carefully documented, in order for the rational choice of any particular surgical procedure to be made.

The fundamental principles of surgical therapy in chronic pancreatitis are the relief of pain and the relief of duct obstruction preventing further pancreatic damage. Ductal distension is widely believed to be an important element in causing pain of chronic pancreatitis, and procedures designed to decompress the pancreatic ducts have been shown successfully to control pain. Decompression of pancreatic ducts may also lead to an improvement in pancreatic function. This is particularly important early in the disease process, as the relief of obstruction is thought to diminish the likelihood of recurrent episodes of acute pancreatitis and stop or delay further pancreatic fibrosis.

A minority of patients with chronic pancreatitis have stenosis or blockage at the Ampulla of Vater. In these cases, pancreatic sphincteroplasty may be of benefit. Correct use of this procedure demands that intrapancreatic duct obstruction be ruled out by ERCP or operative pancreatography. In most patients, generalized duct dilation and multiple strictures are present and these patients may respond to direct pancreatic ductal drainage. An important feature of drainage procedures is the preservation of existing endocrine function by avoidance of pancreatic resection and loss of islet cell mass. Most patients do not require insulin therapy after these operations. The first procedure used to drain the duct system was described by Du Val whereby a loop of jejunum is anastomosed to the distal pancreatic duct forming a distal pancreatico-jejunostomy. The efficacy of this operation, which was frequently complicated by duct blockage, has been improved by Puestow. In this procedure the duct is opened longitudinally and a Roux-en-Y loop of jejunum is anastomosed over this widely opened ductal system (longitudinal pancreatico-jejunostomy). The presence of a large pancreatic cyst may be treated by a cyst-gastrostomy or cyst-jejunostomy.

For disease restricted to either the head or tail of the gland, partial resections may be useful. Distal pancreatectomy is a relatively easy procedure to perform, but in only a minority of all patients with chronic pancreatitis will pain and pancreatic function be improved. Whipple's operation may occasionally be used when the head of the pancreas is involved in the inflammatory process. Frequently this operation is difficult owing to extensive retroperitoneal fibrosis. In most patients, chronic pancreatitis involves the whole gland and, in carefully selected patients, extensive resections have been advocated when duct dilation is absent. The most commonly used major resection procedure is that devised by Child and colleagues known as the 95% distal pancreatectomy. This procedure preserves the stomach, duodenum and distal bile duct and has been quite successful in the control of pain. This operation is superior to total pancreatectomy in that exocrine replacement and nutritional status are more readily controlled. However, resection procedures are accompanied by a significant morbidity and mortality. Patients invariably require insulin to control diabetes. In addition, the patient must remain on total pancreatic replacements for life. The post pancreatectomy diabetic is frequently unstable and requires careful management of diet and insulin therapy. Indeed, deaths from diabetic complications are frequent following pancreatectomy. Despite removal of virtually all the pancreas, some patients still have pain and this can be difficult to control.

In those patients where pain is severe and a direct operative approach is not possible, a variety of procedures are available to control this symptom. These include autonomic splanchnicectomy and coeliac plexus injection. There is good documentation of early control of pain using these procedures although pain frequently recurs after several months.

Surgery for chronic pancreatitis demands careful preoperative selection of patients. Each case must be individually assessed and psychiatric help may be needed to predict further alcohol abuse. Every attempt must be made to conserve pancreatic tissue; thus major resection procedures should be reserved for those patients who fail to respond to simple measures and who will not stop drinking. Surgery for selected patients gives excellent short-term results but the overall long-term benefits are disappointing.

Case 24

A 65-year-old man presented as an emergency when a clinical diagnosis of acute cholecystitis was made Gallstones
had been diagnosed on an ultrasound scan 6 months earlier
when he had mild dyspepia. It was decided to perform a
cholecystectomy as an emergency operation. At operation,
the gallbladder was moderately inflamed, contained biliary
mud but no stones, and an operative cholangiogram showed
no evidence of stones within the bile duct, whose diameter
was 10 mm. Contrast medium passed into the duodenum on
all three films. The gallbladder was removed using retrograde dissection and the patient made an uneventful
recovery. Two months later he developed jaundice with an
obstructive pattern of biochemistry and marked pruritus.

Questions

What is the differential diagnosis?
What investigations should be performed?

Discussion

The most likely diagnosis is that of a retained common bile
duct stone. The patient denied any pain and the operative
cholangiogram was reported as normal. Retained common
bile duct stones producing jaundice usually cause biliary
colic as they become wedged in the upper part of the
sphincter muscle; however, pain is not always present. In
addition, stones can be overlooked at operative cholangiography, particularly when the contrast medium completely
surrounds the stone, thus obscuring it.

The second most likely diagnosis is that the bile duct had
been damaged at the operation. This was felt by the surgeon
to be extremely unlikely as the cystic, common hepatic and
common bile ducts had all been seen clearly at operation
and the gallbladder had been removed retrogradely before
ligating the cystic duct (through which an adequate operative cholangiogram had been performed).

The third possibility is that some additional pathology was

present or had arisen subsequent to the laparotomy. Such pathology could be a carcinoma of the ampulla of Vater, a carcinoma of the head of the pancreas, a cholangiocarcinoma or a hepatocellular carcinoma.

The other possibility is that the patient had developed infectious hepatitis which may have related to his previous hospital admission. He had neither received a blood transfusion nor plasma products; hepatitis A would therefore be more likely than hepatitis B, the incubation period for the former being about 2 months.

The investigations which are appropriate are: bilirubin 360 mmol/l, ALT 48 U/l, alkaline phosphatase 1,018 U/l. Hepatitis B surface antigen was negative and there was no elevation in α-fetoprotein. Ultrasound scan of the liver and biliary tree showed a dilated common bile duct and intrahepatic biliary radicles. An ERCP was performed which confirmed complete occlusion at the lower end of the common bile duct and in addition the pancreatic duct was totally occluded near to the ampulla.

The patient was shown to have a carcinoma of the head of the pancreas, about 1.5 cm in diameter. It is probable that this tumour had produced the patient's acute cholecystitis but re-examination of the common bile duct on the initial operative cholangiogram showed no abnormality.

This case was eminently suitable for a Whipple's operation. The tumour was small and apparently confined to the head of the pancreas without having invaded the portal vein, hepatic artery or adjacent lymph nodes. Whilst this operation has a mortality rate of about 20%, it offers the only hope of cure in this condition. Also, whilst the overall 5-year survival rate is less than 1% for carcinoma of the pancreas in those with small tumours which satisfy the above criteria, the rate of survival at five years may approach 20%.

For the vast majority of patients with carcinoma of the head of the pancreas palliative by-pass is all that can be offered to relieve the patient's jaundice. Cholecystojejunostomy, jejunojejunostomy and sometimes gastroenterostomy is the usual form of by-pass carried out, and results in resolution of jaundice, with a survival period often reaching 1 to 2 years. Radiotherapy and chemotherapy have little established role in the treatment of carcinoma of the pancreas.

Case 25

A 37-year-old woman presented with a history of midline epigastric pain and weight loss. The boring pain was exacerbated by food and relieved by lying prone; there was direct posterior radiation to the upper lumbar region. Abdominal examination revealed no abnormality. Barium meal and follow-through examination, endoscopy, barium enema, serum amylase, urea, electrolytes and liver function tests were all normal. The haemoglobin concentration was 11.7 g/dl. Upper abdominal ultrasound suggested a mass lesion in the region of the pancreatic neck; this was confirmed using CT.

Questions

How may the diagnosis be obtained?
What treatment is available?
What is the prognosis for this condition?

Discussion

A tissue diagnosis of a pancreatic mass may be obtained on ultrasound, by laparoscopy, at ERCP examination or at laparotomy. A fine needle can be guided under ultrasound control into the pancreatic mass and cytological examination of the aspirate is carried out. At laparoscopy, the tumour can be visualised and biopsied through a separate 'stab wound' in the abdomen. The liver can also be inspected. An ERCP examination will allow visualization of the pancreatic duct. The pancreatic fluid may be collected for cytology and brushings can be obtained from the duct. Laparotomy was chosen in this case for the following reasons: (i) it provided the only way of accurately assessing the tumour and its local extent; (ii) it allowed accurate assessment of the lymphatic spread and more detailed inspection of the liver and *porta hepatis;* (iii) it obviated the risk of dissemination of the tumour by the methods described above; (iv) it permitted more accurate tissue sampling for biopsy when the tumour was surrounded by chronic inflammation, and (v) it allowed the appropriate surgical treatment to be carried out at the earliest opportunity. The disadvantage of performing a laparotomy before a tissue diagnosis has been made is that the incorrect diagnosis may be made from macroscopic examination of the pancreas at operation. In addition, the interpretation of frozen section specimens of the pancreas can be difficult. Conversely, more accurate biopsy can be taken at operation and since pancreatic neoplasms are often surrounded by areas of chronic pancreatitis the exact sample taken is of utmost importance. The combined sensitivity and specificity of an accurate, large tissue biopsy obtained at laparotomy must thus be superior to the sample obtained by needle biopsy. This approach was therefore used in the above reported case, and the tissue was reported as a poorly differentiated carcinoma of the pancreas. The histological diagnosis was confirmed on the paraffin sections. If hepatic scans using ultrasound or CT show tumour, then needle biopsy of the tumour tissue within the liver should be carried out.

The treatment of carcinoma of the body of the pancreas is very disappointing both in terms of reasonable palliation and long-term survival. Overall, for cancer of the exocrine pancreas, the 5-year survival rate is less than 5%. All of these survivors had disease which was confined to the pancreatic head and presented with obstructive jaundice prior to the occurrence of extrapancreatic spread. Carcinoma of the body and tail of the pancreas only becomes clinically manifest when the disease has spread outside the confines of the pancreas to invade adjacent organs. There are no 5-year survivors in patients with tumours in these situations; however, it is usual, where technically possible, to excise the tumour by performing a distal pancreatectomy. This may provide pain relief but there is no evidence that it improves long-term survival. Pain relief may also be achieved by injecting the splanchnic nerves or coeliac ganglion with a sclerosing agent such as ethanol (50%) or phenol (6%). There is no established role for radiotherapy in the treatment of carcinoma of the body of the pancreas, although a trial is now being performed in Boston of the use of peroperative radiotherapy applied locally at the time of open operation. Chemotherapy is capable of producing a measurable therapeutic response in terms of tumour regression: 5-fluouracil 28%; mitomycin C 27%; methyl CCNU 13%; streptozotocin 11-

36% and adriamycin 13%. Combination chemotherapy may produce a greater response; however, none of these agents, either individually or in combination, has been shown to substantially prolong life and their morbidity is considerable. The combination of radiotherapy with chemotherapy may hold some promise, as suggested by the results of one study combining 5-fluouracil with 6000 rads given via an external beam.

For most patients with advanced pancreatic cancer all that can be offered is supportive therapy in the form of pain relief, ultimately using opiates. Institutionalization in an appropriate hospice can be valuable for both patients and their families.

Case 26

A 24-year-old joiner presented with a 1-year history of pain in the right iliac fossa associated with some pain in the region of the right hip. His symptoms had been virtually continuous over this period but were slowly becoming more severe. Over the weeks prior to presentation, exacerbations of lower abdominal colic had been associated with abdominal distension and borborygmi. Occasionally, the pain had radiated directly through to his back. During the course of his illness the patient had lost four stones in weight and had been subject to intermittent bouts of diarrhoea. A further symptom was marked anorexia, the patient being unable to face the sight or smell of food. There was no history of dermatological problems, joint pains, eye or urinary symptoms. On examination, he appeared cachectic and a large firm and fixed mass was present in his right iliac fossa extending across the midline and apparent on rectal examination. There was no evidence of perianal disease.

The haemoglobin concentration was 11.2 g/dl, white cell count $17.4 \times 10^9/l$ and erythrocyte sedimentation rate of 68 mm in the first hour. Electrolyte concentration and liver function tests were normal with the exception of an elevated alkaline phosphatase (342 U/l).

Questions

What is the most likely diagnosis?
What is the differential diagnosis?
What treatment is indicated?
What is the prognosis?

Discussion

A barium enema showed a normal colon with the exception of the caecum which was irregular and deformed. Only a small amount of contrast medium entered the terminal ileum which appeared strictured. A barium meal and follow-through showed a string sign of Kantor in the terminal ileum with rose thorn ulceration characteristic of Crohn's disease. There was some narrowing of the distal aspect of the second part of the duodenum also suggestive of Crohn's disease.

The differential diagnosis includes tuberculosis, carcinoma of the caecum, small intestinal lymphoma, non-specific terminal ileitis, eosinophitic gastroenteritis and campylobacter enteritis. A rectal biopsy is often helpful in making the diagnosis of Crohn's disease, where granulomata are present in the mucosa.

The management of uncomplicated ileal Crohn's disease should be conservative, supportive and non-operative. A nutritious high protein diet is to be recommended with supplements of iron, folate, Vitamin B12, Vitamin D and zinc. A medium chain triglyceride diet has been recommended. Prednisolone (20-60 mg daily) has been shown to be effective in abating the severe flare up of the disease. Salazopyrin (up to 1 g q.d.s.) has a place in the conservative management of colonic Crohn's disease, but is of questionable value in small intestinal disease. It has been shown in a recent study that patients receiving adrenocorticotrophic hormone (ACTH) fared better than those given oral corticosteroids. Occasionally patients respond to treatment with azathioprine; these are in a minority but the response can be dramatic. In addition sporadic cases respond to metronidazole, and this is of most value in treating perianal disease.

Sodium cromoglycate and levamisole have been investigated but lack any firm scientific evidence in their favour.

The course of the disease can be serially monitored using an activity index, a system of scoring according to clinical, biochemical and radiological factors.

Operative treatment is reserved for the complications of the disease and for disease progression despite medical treatment. The indications for surgery are: (i) intestinal obstruction; (ii) failure to respond to medical therapy; (iii) fistula formation; (iv) abscess formation; (v) toxic dilatation of the colon; and (vi) perianal complications. The vast majority of cases will require surgical treatment during the course of the disease.

In this case, a right hemicolectomy was performed with excision of the involved terminal ileum. The principles of surgical treatment are: (i) as much normal bowel as possible must be conserved; (ii) strictures and fistulae should be resected to macroscopically normal areas of bowel on each side; (iii) meticulous care must be exercised in performing anastomoses; (iv) exclusion bypass should be avoided; (v) proximal ileostomy may be useful; resection may be limited to the obstructed segment of bowel when most, or all of the small bowel is involved; and where multiple short strictures exist these may be widened by a plastic procedure.

Intravenous feeding may be helpful both pre- and post-operatively.

The incidence of recurrent Crohn's disease in such a young patient is considerable, probably amounting to at least 75%. The mortality rate associated with the condition is not high, and overall accounts for about twice that expected from the normal age and sex-matched control population.

Case 27

A 52-year-old man presented with a 3-year history of diarrhoea and 2 years of flushing attacks during which he stated that his whole body became 'red'. He had more recently developed chest pain and breathlessness associated with a 'blue' discolouration of his face and hands. In addition, he complained of upper abdominal and right hypochondrial discomfort. Mild exercise or the slightest stress exacerbated his symptoms of flushing and on some occasions produced vertigo. The diarrhoea had been improved by a kaolin and morphine mixture and by aluminium hydroxide.

There was a past history of myocardial infarctions occurring at the age of 37 and 42 years; at that time he had been a heavy smoker.

On examination he was markedly plethoric. The lung fields were clear. He had a loud systolic murmur over the precordium characteristic of a pulmonary flow murmur. The liver was enlarged, particularly in the epigastrium where a discrete mass could be palpated. There was no evidence of ascites, but mild peripheral oedema was present.

Questions

What is the likely diagnosis?
What investigations are indicated?
What is the treatment?

Discussion

This patient has the clinical features of the carcinoid syndrome. The student might find the mnemonic A–F of help: ascites, breathlessness, cyanosis, diarrhoea, oedema and flushing.

Ultrasound of the abdomen demonstrated multiple focal echogenic lesions in the liver, in keeping with metastatic deposits of carcinoid tumour. Chest X-ray showed no abnormality in the lung fields, but there was some cardiac enlargement. Barium meal and follow-through and barium enema examinations were both normal. The 24-hour urinary output of 5-hydroxy-indole-acetic acid (5 HIAA) was 2625 μmol. Selectivity coeliac axis arteriography showed that the common hepatic artery arose normally from the coeliac axis, and demonstrated a diffuse tumour circulation with the liver substance. CT also showed the presence of multiple metastases, the disease appeared to be confined to the liver.

Laparotomy revealed a small primary neoplasm in the caecum with multiple lymphnode metastases in the mesentery. The liver was largely replaced by metastatic deposits. A right hemicolectomy was performed and the common hepatic artery was ligated. The 5 HIAA output was approximately halved by the operation and remained at a level of approximately 1200 μmol for 6 months, but thereafter began to increase. One year after his operation the patient became severely incapacitated by flushing attacks, and was subsequently treated with chemotherapy.

The fundamental treatment of carcinoid tumours is surgical; wherever possible the primary tumor should be excised. Following excision of a discrete appendicular primary, which is usually benign, few tumours will give rise to further problems. Primary tumours of the caecum and small intestine are much more likely to be malignant and to metastasize. For advanced metastatic disease involving the liver, arterial embolization or ligation is the treatment of choice, both radiotherapy and chemotherapy have proved disappointing in their therapeutic effect.

Patients with a well established carcinoid syndrome should be advised to abstain from alcohol, heavy exercise and certain foodstuffs which the patient finds produce his symptoms. Cardiac failure may require treatment and codeine phosphate is helpful for diarrhoea; potassium supplements may also be required. Methyldopa may reduce the catecholamine stimulated release of flush-producing substances and parachlorophenylalanine (1g q.d.s.) has been shown to block the enzyme that converts tryptophan to 5-hydroxytryptamine. Methysergide, cyproheptadine and ketanserin have been used as 5-hydroxytryptamine antagonists with moderate success.

Case 28

A 63-year-old man presented with intermittent claudication involving predominantly the left leg, after several further months he developed pain in the right leg when at rest. The patient had been a heavy smoker of cigarettes for many years and had hypercholesterolaemia which was being treated with clofibrate (Atromid-S). Arteriography showed complete occlusion of the right common iliac artery with a tight stenosis of the left common iliac artery. The terminal aorta was almost completely occluded by atheroma. Both of the superficial femoral and profunda femoris arteries were widely patent. A Cooley double velour aortic bifurcation graft was inserted dividing the aorta transversely and performing an end-to-side anastomosis to both common femoral arteries.

Following an uneventful recovery he was discharged on the twelfth postoperative day, but later developed a cold, pale right leg and was readmitted 3 weeks after his surgery. The graft was explored through the right groin where a plaque of atheroma at the anastomosis had apparently produced a thrombosis of the right limb of the graft. The thrombus was removed and the circulation restored. One month later, he again developed rest pain in the right leg and there was thrombosis of the right limb of the graft along with the common femoral artery and the origins of the superficial femoral and profunda femoris arteries. The aortic bifurcation graft was removed and a further graft was inserted, following which the patient developed an abdominal wound infection, but then made a good recovery.

He remained well for 3 years and was able to walk several miles without developing claudication. The patient next developed an iron deficient anaemia with a haemoglobin concentration of 6.1 g/dl, faecal occult blood estimations were consistently strongly positive.

Questions

What investigations are indicated?
What is the treatment of choice?

Discussion

Gastroduodenoscopy showed no abnormality and colonoscopy was also normal, as was barium meal, follow-through examination and barium enema. Ultrasound of the aortic bifurcation graft showed no abnormality. No source of bleeding could be identified on selective coeliac and mesenteric arteriography or on isotope studies using radiolabelled red cells. The patient continued to bleed and laparotomy was performed.

No abnormality was apparent in the gastrointestinal tract until the third part of the duodenum was inspected. Careful mobilization of the duodenum amidst dense adhesions revealed that the upper end of the aortic bifurcation graft was heavily stained with bile. Further mobilization revealed a small full-thickness defect in the duodenum, the aorta appeared intact. The features were those of an aorto-duodenal fistula, with intermittent blood loss occurring into the duodenum from the infected aortic suture line.

The third part of the duodenum was resected and reanastomosed; the anastomosis was then separated from the aorta by a plug of omentum which was placed around the aorta.

The patient was treated with long-term antibiotics (Augmentin and metronidazole) and remained well for 2 years. He then again became anaemic, faecal occult blood estimations once more being consistently positive. Investigations for the source of blood loss again proved negative, it was assumed to be due to a recurrent aorto-duodenal fistula. The possibility of excising the bifurcation graft and carrying out axillo-bifemoral grafts was considered, but at that time the patient was found to have bony metastases from a hypernephroma. In view of this and his poor general condition, a conservative policy was pursued with continued antibiotic therapy. The patient finally developed a major haemorrhage from his aorto-duodenal fistula and died two-and-a-half years after the operation was performed for his fistula.

The commonly recommended treatment of an aorto-duodenal fistula is excision of the infected graft and the performance of axillo-bifemoral grafts. This was not performed in the present case because of the patient's poor general condition, the relatively low femoral anastomosis following the revised aortic bifurcation graft and the consequent risk of impaired rectal viability. The more conservative approach employed would render complete eradication of sepsis in relation to the aortic anastomosis virtually impossible. When prosthetic material at any site in the body becomes infected the chances of eradicating the infection by the use of broad spectrum antibiotics are almost non-existent. The only possible way of overcoming the infective process is to remove the graft and to insert any further prosthetic material in an anatomical site which is separate from the initial one.

Whilst the performance of axillo-bifemoral grafts is not, in itself, a major operation, removal of the infected graft material is, and the risks of ischaemia to the pelvic tissues is considerable. It was hoped that the interposition of omentum between the aorta and the duodenum might prevent further fistula formation and this was the case for two years. When recurrent bleeding occurred, death was imminent from an unrelated cause, that of widespread metastases from a hypernephroma.

Case 29

A 63-year-old man presented with abdominal pain of sudden onset. The pain was situated across the central abdomen and, whilst initially mild, had increased in severity, being continuously present with little fluctuation in its intensity. Soon after the onset of pain he developed an urge to defaecate, the stools appearing normal. The patient had atrial fibrillation, there was little abdominal tenderness and no other intra-abdominal abnormality.

Investigations showed a leucocytosis of $15.7 \times 10^9/l$ and a mild metabolic acidosis. The serum amylase was elevated at 620 U/l. There was a slight elevation of the serum phosphate concentration (1.6 mmol/l). Chest X-ray showed no abnormality but an electrocardiogram revealed atrial fibrillation.

Questions

What is the differential diagnosis?
What further investigations may be helpful?
How should the patient be treated?

Discussion

The diagnosis here was acute mesenteric vascular occlusion which is notoriously difficult to diagnose in its early stages, but for optimal success with treatment early diagnosis is mandatory. The differential diagnosis lies between: acute pancreatitis, acute intestinal obstruction, acute cholecystitis, acute appendicitis, an exacerbation of a peptic ulcer, volvulus or intussusception involving the small bowel. A definite clue to the diagnosis is the history of atrial fibrillation which predisposes to the production of intra-atrial thrombus. This then becomes detached and produces an embolus, usually lodging close to the origin of the superior mesenteric artery just distal to the first branch, namely the inferior pancreatico-duodenal artery. Most commonly the embolus only partially obstructs the artery.

Further investigations which might be helpful when superior mesenteric arterial occlusion is suspected are laparoscopy, angiography, isotope scanning and ultrasound. Laparoscopy is safe, simple, quick to perform and may reveal the classical appearances of dusky bowel and turbid intraperitoneal fluid. Selective superior mesenteric angiography may be used to identify the lesion and, in addition, show those with a surgically correctable occlusion and those with diffuse vascular spasm. Early angiography has been advocated in those over the age of 50 years developing sudden and severe, otherwise unexplained abdominal pain with a known predisposing factor such as atrial fibrillation. Several radiopharmaceuticals have been investigated experimentally: 99 m TC pyrophosphate, diphosphonate or labelled leucocytes, in the hope that they might be taken up by the ischaemic bowel. Their clinical role has not yet been established. Ultrasound scanning may reveal a dissecting aneurysm producing occlusion of the superior mesenteric artery. Doppler ultrasound is being developed to detect mesenteric occlusion and to measure mesenteric blood flow. The elevation of serum phosphate may be significant and acts as an indicator to this diagnosis.

In the management of this condition initial full assessment of the patient is essential. Associated cardiovascular problems, particularly congestive cardiac failure and cardiac arrhythmias, are treated and the blood volume restored. Low molecular weight Dextran should be given since it acts both as a plasma expander and in decreasing platelet adhesiveness. Broad spectrum antibiotics should be administered to control any tendency for septicaemia occurring from non-viable mucosa. Cefoxitin or a combination of metronidazole and netilmicin are appropriate. If the urinary output is low, mannitol or frusemide should be given. Anticoagulants have no proven role in the management of the condition.

Surgery is indicated when the patient develops signs of peritonism or where a major degree of occlusion exists on selective angiography. Two therapeutic options exist: embolectomy and resection, or both. Embolectomy should be attempted in the early stages of the disorder when there is a possibility of some of the ischaemic bowel regaining viability, and is best performed by a direct approach close to the origin of the vessel. The embolus is removed and Fogarty catheters are passed along the vessel. The viability of the bowel may visibly improve but a 'second look' laparotomy is to be recommended 12 to 24 hours later. Where short segments of non-viable bowel are present these should be resected. The use of a temporary ileostomy will overcome the risk of dehiscence of a non-viable anastomosis. More extensive segments of ischaemic bowel should be treated by removal of the worst portions followed by a 'second look' laparotomy 12 to 24 hours later.

If there is total occlusion of the superior mesenteric artery and the diagnosis has been delayed, infarction occurs from the proximal 30-45 cm of jejunum round to the right side of the colon or the proximal transverse colon. If the patient's condition is stable enough to warrant it, resection of all the non-viable bowel should be carried out. A small proportion of these patients may maintain adequate nutrition orally with dietary supplements but long-term parenteral nutrition may be required. The mortality following a major vascular occlusion is of the order of 80%.

Case 30

A 26-year-old patient presented with a two-year history of abdominal pain associated with diarrhoea and weight loss.

Investigations confirmed the presence of Crohn's disease of the distal jejunum and proximal ileum. He underwent small bowel resection with primary anastomosis. No other evidence of small bowel Crohn's syndrome was identified. Pathological investigation of the resected specimen revealed one end to be involved with microscopic areas of Crohn's disease. Postoperatively, the patient initially made good progress but on the sixth postoperative day frank small bowel contents discharged through the drain. The next three days this turned into a high output small bowel fistula with greater than one litre of small bowel content draining per day.

Investigations

At the time of fistula formation the biochemistry was as follows: Haemoglobin 9.5 g/dl, white count $20.6 \times 10^9/l$, urea 16.5 mmol/l, sodium 128 mmol/l, potassium 2.7 mmol/l and albumin 29 g/l.

Questions

Discuss the pathology of small bowel fistulae.
How should this patient be managed?

Discussion

Small bowel fistulae occurring in the postoperative period are almost always resultant on anastomotic leakage although occasionally a peritoneal abscess can penetrate the bowel or an inadvertently placed suture may erode into the bowel. These fistulae usually present through the drainage site or the main incision. They are often heralded by the presence of abdominal pain, pyrexia and abdominal distension. Anastomotic leakage may result from poor surgical technique, poor blood flow at the anastomotic site, the presence of disease at one side of the anastomosis (as in this patient) and the presence of localised infection.

Patients with Crohn's disease are particularly prone to fistulae, thus great care must be taken during surgery. It is important to localise the site of fistula formation, although this should be apparent from the previous anastomosis. A Gastrografin or barium meal and follow-through can be performed which will show the site of fistula formation and whether contrast material enters the distal bowel. Evidence of distal obstruction may also be shown.

The mainstays of treatment in these patients are firstly, to prevent oral intake. This will reduce the secretion in the biliary and pancreatic trees and also within the small bowel itself. Intravenous fluid should then be administered. These patients, as in this case, are frequently dehydrated with concomitant electrolyte imbalance which requires correction. Parenteral nutrition must be considered in all patients with a high output fistula or evidence of severe malnutrition as in this patient with anaemia and hypoalbuminaemia. Parenteral nutrition should be instituted through a carefully placed central venous line which should be tunnelled subcutaneously to prevent catheter sepsis. Three litres of fluid per day should be administered, and this should contain fat, protein and carbohydrates. Added vitamins and electrolytes should also be given. Additional crystalloids are usually needed to compensate for electrolyte loss in the fistulous fluid.

The site of the fistula itself must be also carefully assessed. This fistulous fluid will contain digestive enzymes and thus careful skin protection is essential to obviate the distressing sequelae of dermatitis and ulceration. The skin should be protected by barrier creams and careful bag application is frequently required to allow collection of the fluid. The fluid volume must be carefully monitored and correlated with urine output and the volume of parenteral nutrition given. With this management, there is often a gradual reduction in the quantity of the fistulous discharge until eventually the fistula closes.

In some situations, a small bowel fistula will not close spontaneously. There are several reasons for this, mainly, distal obstruction of the small bowel, a total discontinuity of the bowel ends, an associated abscess cavity with localised infection and the presence of disease within the small bowel itself such as malignancy or Crohn's disease.

This patient was managed by reducing oral intake to zero and parenteral nutrition was instituted. The skin was carefully protected and the fluid collected. After 2 weeks of therapy, his fistulous output remained at 1 l/day although his blood indices and clinical state were much improved. Barium meal and follow through performed at this stage showed the fistula to be at the site of anastomosis with evidence of distal obstruction.

It was decided that operation was necessary and this was performed one week later when his clinical condition had optimally improved.

The old laparotomy wound was excised and the fistulous track carefully dissected out. An extra 20 cm of small bowel was resected on either side of the previous anastomosis and a further small bowel anastomosis performed. A small intraperitoneal abscess, associated with this, was also drained.

Following this procedure, the patient made a slow but steady recovery. Parenteral nutrition was discontinued at 5 weeks and, following this, the patient tolerated oral fluids and food normally. He was discharged from hospital 9 weeks after the original operation; the value of parenteral nutrition was illustrated by his weight remaining virtually the same as on presentation.

Case 31

A 62-year-old woman presented with a 4-day history of abdominal pain associated with vomiting, constipation and abdominal distension. This pain appeared to be colicky in nature and was related to profuse vomiting.

Her past medical history included an appendicectomy performed 23 years previously and an abdominal hysterectomy performed 5 years previously.

On examination, she was dehydrated with loss of skin elasticity and sunken eyeballs. There was no evidence of anaemia or pyrexia. Abdominal examination revealed marked distension but no evidence of peritonitis. Areas of tenderness were found in the lower part of the abdomen and bowel sounds were increased and high-pitched. These bowel sounds were particularly associated with episodes of pain. Rectal examination was unremarkable. Vaginal examination was normal considering the previous hysterectomy.

Investigations

Haemoglobin 16.3 g/dl, white count $12.3 \times 10^9/l$, urea 17.8 mmol/l, sodium 128 mmol/l, potassium 2.9 mmol/l, bicarbonate 26 mmol/l, albumin 35 g/l. Chest X-ray was normal with no evidence of gas under the diaphragm. Supine abdominal X-ray revealed marked distension of the small bowel with no evidence of gas in the large bowel. Erect films demonstrated multiple small bowel fluid levels.

Questions

Discuss the pathology of small bowel obstruction.
How should this patient be managed?

Discussion

Small bowel obstruction may be either mechanical or adynamic in the presence of paralytic ileus. Mechanical small bowel obstruction, as in this patient, may be simple or related to strangulation. In simple obstruction the main feature is distension of the bowel proximal to the obstructing lesion. Distension is related to the presence of increased quantities of gas within the small bowel. Most of this gas comes from swallowed air with small amounts coming from bacteria within the gut and direct transfer from the blood. Nasogastric tubes will control most of the gaseous distension, thus confirming the importance of swallowed air in producing this effect. Large quantities of fluid also present within the gut are related to gastrointestinal secretions and ingested fluids. Normally 8-10 l of secretions enter the gut per day and all but 100/200 ml are reabsorbed. These fluids are a solution of electrolytes, and loss of them results in a direct drain on extracellular fluid. Within the first 6 hours of obstruction there is decreased absorption from the gut after which there is an increase in secretion. A combination of decreased absorption and increased secretion from the gut results in large quantities of fluid being present within the small bowel. With low small bowel obstruction several litres of fluid can be lost within the gut.

The presence of small bowel obstruction also results in multiplication of bacteria within the obstructed segment. These bacteria, which include coliforms, faecal streptococci and anaerobic organisms, produce toxins which are absorbed and thus play a part in the illness of intestinal obstruction. The toxins may be absorbed through the blood, the lymphatics and probably, most importantly, through the peritoneum. The presence of gut distension results in an increase in intraluminal pressure within the small bowel. Normally, the pressure within the small bowel is within the range of 2-4 mmHg. In the presence of obstruction, the pressure within the small bowel rises to values of greater than 10 mmHg. Bowel distension initially results in an increase in peristaltic activity which causes a tense colicky pain, although later paresis ensues. Impaired viability of the bowel eventually occurs resulting in perforation.

Strangulation obstruction is a particularly serious condition as blood loss occurs due to venous blockage and later arterial obstruction. Indeed, with large lengths of bowel a considerable amount of blood can be lost within the strangulated segment. Furthermore, strangulation results in marked toxaemia with a peritoneal exudate of bacteria and red blood cells.

The classical clinical features of small bowel obstruction are those of vomiting, intestinal colic, distension and constipation. High small bowel obstruction is usually associated with marked vomiting and little distension; conversely, low obstruction produces the opposite symptoms. Abdominal ascultation in patients with mechanical obstruction will reveal periods of increasing, high-pitched or tinkling bowel sounds separated by relatively quiet periods. Rectal examination should be performed in every case to detect luminal and extraluminal pathology. Faeces, if present, should be tested for occult blood which may indicate carcinoma, intussusception or infarction.

Careful initial management of patients with bowel obstruction is vital. As in this patient, urea and electrolyte estimations frequently demonstrate marked hyponatraemia, hypokalaemia and a raised urea secondary to the loss of fluid and electrolytes from the gut. An intravenous line must be placed and the fluid and electrolyte imbalance corrected. This may require large volumes of saline and dextrose solutions with added potassium. In addition, a nasogastric tube is passed to relieve distension and prevent vomiting. In patients with marked fluid loss, a urinary catheter is useful in assessing fluid balance. Pain relief must be given in the form of opiates.

Strangulation obstruction is a surgical emergency, and these patients also require parenteral antibiotics and blood or plasma in addition to the above measures. In this clinical situation, where there is evidence of peritonitis, toxaemia or a visible obstruction (e.g. hernia), early operation is mandatory. This early operative intervention may prevent irreversible strangulation from occurring and obviate small bowel resection. In patients where there is no evidence of strangulation, a conservative early policy should be adopted. If there are signs of definite improvement, then emergency surgery may be avoided.

Small bowel obstruction in the United Kingdom is frequently related to adhesions, and is the most likely diagnosis in this patient. Such obstruction may settle spontaneously on a conservative management of 'drip and suck', in which case no surgery is needed. Other causes of small bowel obstruction must be excluded by careful examination; these include herniae, (femoral, inguinal, incisional and umbilical) and carcinoma (primary and secondary). Rarer causes of obstruction include gallstone ileus with gas in the biliary tree on abdominal X-ray, Crohn's disease, internal herniae, radiation, food bolus, intussusception, intestinal infarction due to mesenteric vein thrombosis or artery embolism/thrombosis and volvulus.

The patient with suspected adhesive small bowel obstruction should undergo surgery when pulse, blood-pressure, urinary output and blood electrolytes are normal. Operation in the absence of external hernia should be performed through a midline or paramedian incision. A careful laparotomy is performed and the site of bowel obstruction determined. Adhesive bands are then divided and the entire small bowel cleared of obstruction. When there is doubt about intestinal viability, the bowel should be completely released and placed in warm packs for 5 minutes and then re-examined. If normal colour has returned and peristalsis is evident, it is safe to return the bowel. Non-viable or doubtful bowel must be resected with primary small bowel anastomosis. In this patient, the small bowel was dilated down to the distal ileum and obstruction was caused by adhesions in the pelvis related to the previous hysterectomy. The adhesions were divided and the bowel was viable. When bowel distension is very marked, operative decompression can be performed using a Savage decompressor. In situations of repeated small bowel obstruction related to adhesions, a Noble's plication operation can be attempted to prevent further trouble.

Case 32

A 72-year-old woman presented with a 3-day history of increasing abdominal pain, distension and vomiting, she had been seen by a general practitioner on two occasions and diagnosed as having gastroenteritis. There was no relevant past medical history.

On admission to hospital she was found to be very dehydrated with a blood pressure of 90/60 mmHg and a pulse of 140/min. Examination of the abdomen revealed marked distension with evidence of peritonitis and absent bowel sounds. Rectal examination was unremarkable. In the right groin there was a lump 5 cm in diameter just below the inguinal ligament which was extremely tender to palpation.

Investigations

Sodium 128 mmol/l, potassium 2.6 mmol/l, urea 27.3 mmol/l, haemoglobin 10.9 g/dl, white count 17.3 × 10^9/l, creatinine 336 μmol/l. The chest X-ray was normal, but abdominal X-rays showed evidence of small bowel distension with numerous fluid levels.

Questions

What is the diagnosis in this patient?
How should she be best managed in the peri-operative period.?

Discussion

This patient is extremely ill as a result of an untreated, probable strangulated femoral hernia. As she was shocked and had evidence of septicaemia, she required careful pre-operative resuscitation. This consisted of the insertion of an intravenous fluid line and a nasogastric tube. Initially, she was given two units of plasma; this was followed by crystalloid infusion with saline containing potassium supplements. A urinary catheter was then passed and the patient was given broad spectrum antibiotics, (metronidazole and gentamicin). Pethidine was also given for pain relief. Because of their narrow necks, femoral herniae have a particular propensity for strangulation. In some cases, only part of the bowel is trapped and this forms a Richter's hernia. After 4 hours of resuscitation, the present patient's blood pressure and pulse had returned to normal levels and her urine output was satisfactory. The operation was performed through a lower right pararectal incision (McEvedy's approach). A large femoral hernia was found with a tight neck which could not be easily reduced. Peritonitis was present, resulting from contamination by small bowel contents. A loop of small bowel had become trapped within the femoral hernia and, after reduction, this was found to be black and necrotic, with a perforation causing peritonitis. The hernia itself could only be reduced by dividing the lacunar ligament, and 2 feet of small bowel was resected with end-to-end anastomosis. The peritoneal cavity was carefully cleaned and irrigated with antibiotic solution. The femoral canal was closed with a loose suture of prolene, care being taken not to encroach upon the femoral vein. Postoperatively, the patient developed a profound paralytic ileus; however, this gradually resolved and she was able to tolerate all fluids by the seventh postoperative day. She was discharged 15 days postoperatively.

Femoral herniae are more common in women than men; nevertheless, inguinal herniae remain the more common groin hernia in women. A much greater percentage of femoral herniae present as an emergency when compared to inguinal herniae. This is related to their narrow neck, since the femoral canal itself is small and bounded by the inguinal ligament, the lacunar ligament, the pectineal ligament and the femoral vein. Operation in the elective phase may be easily performed with a low surgical approach. In an acute emergency, a higher incision should be used and those approaches described by McEvedy and Lothiessen are probably the best. With these incisions the peritoneal cavity can easily be opened, the viability of the bowel inspected and bowel resection carried out if necessary. With the presence of peritonitis, care must be taken to perform adequate peritoneal toilet and the use of antibiotic solutions has been shown to be very effective in preventing postoperative sepsis. Again emphasis must be placed on the importance of examining the groins in all patients with an acute abdomen, as a small hernia can be easily missed, especially in the obese patient.

Case 33

A 46-year-old man presented with a 1-year history of iron deficiency anaemia. This was associated with frequent abdominal cramps and occasional distension and vomiting. On examination, the patient was clinically anaemic. There were no signs of lymphadenopathy and abdominal examination was unremarkable. Rectal examination was normal although the stools were positive/occult blood testing.

Investigations

Haemoglobin 8.5 g/dl, MCV 68.2 fl. Occult bloods positive. Chemistry normal. Chest X-ray and plain abdominal X-ray normal. Gastroscopy normal. Barium meal and follow through normal. Sigmoidoscopy, colonoscopy and barium enema all normal.

Questions

What further investigations should this patient have and what is the likely diagnosis?
Discuss the management of patients with small bowel tumours.

Discussion

This patient has blood loss into the gastrointestinal tract resulting in severe anaemia. The results of multiple investigations, which have all been negative, suggest that the bleeding point is occult and may be related to small bowel pathology. The differential diagnosis of such occult bleeding should include Crohn's disease, angiodysplasia, small bowel tumours (both benign and malignant), arteriovenous malformations and Meckel's diverticulum.

Further investigations should be performed; these include a small bowel enema and angiography. The former investigation allows a more careful examination of the small bowel mucosa and in this patient an abnormality in the upper jejunum, was identified just distal to the ligament of Treitz. Angiography may demonstrate an arteriovenous malformation or tumour circulation in the small bowel. Technetium scanning may be of benefit in excluding a Meckel's diverticulum and the value of radio labelled red blood cells has yet to be proven. Frequently, however, the diagnosis is only made at laparotomy.

In this case, a tumour was found in the upper jejunum corresponding to the abnormality on small bowel enema. The liver and the rest of the small bowel were normal although lymph nodes at the base of the mesentery appeared to be enlarged. The patient underwent small bowel resection with primary anastomosis. Pathology on the resected specimen revealed an adenocarcinoma infiltrating through the serosa with metastatic tumour present within the lymph nodes.

Small bowel tumours are uncommon, which is perhaps

surprising considering the enormous amount of epithelium at risk. Indeed, the reason for their rarity, compared with the stomach and large bowel, has yet to be explained. This rarity often delays the diagnosis as the possibility of a small bowel tumour is often not considered until the disease process is advanced. Regrettably, therefore, these tumours are often diagnosed after metastases to the lymph nodes and liver have already occurred and, in such cases, curative operations cannot be performed. Benign tumours present within the small bowel are relatively more common.

Four main varieties of malignant tumour are found within the small bowel: namely, adenocarcinoma, lymphoma, carcinoid and leiomyosarcoma. Adenocarcinomas are more often found in the duodenum and upper jejunum, as found in the patient described. When present within the ileum, they may be related to the presence of Crohn's disease. Lymphomas are randomly distributed throughout the small bowel. They are non-Hodgkin's in type and may complicate coeliac disease. Benign carcinoid tumours are found most commonly within the appendix; the ileum, in contrast, is the most common site for the malignant variety. The tumours themselves are submucosal in origin, and often the adjacent bowel has an ischaemic appearance suggesting release of local vasoactive peptides. Twenty-five per cent of carcinoids are multiple and metastases may occur to the liver resulting in the carcinoid syndrome. These tumours, although often of great size, are slow-growing, and the patient may live for many years despite the presence of multiple metastases. Leiomyosarcomas occur randomly throughout the small bowel.

Small bowel tumours are often asymptomatic until advanced disease is present. They may result in obstruction either by complete blockage or by intussusception. Bleeding may also occur and this is more common when adenocarcinoma is present. Weight loss is frequent, and lymphomas of the small bowel are prone to perforation. Indeed, physical deterioration in a patient with coeliac disease who is on a strict gluten-free diet, suggests the development of a lymphoma.

At the time of operation more than 50% of carcinomas of the small bowel have metastasized; despite this, however, they should be resected. No adjuvant therapy has been proven to be of value.

Lymphomas should also be resected and further treatment using radiotherapy or chemotherapy should be considered. The 5-year survival rate for small bowel adenocarcinoma is approximately 10-20%. With carcinoid tumours, 70% of patients are alive at 5 years, indeed 20% of patients with hepatic metastases live for more than 5 years.

The patient described made a good recovery from his operation, but re-presented 6 months later with small bowel obstruction. At operation, it was found that he had widespread peritoneal carcinomatosis affecting the upper small bowel and no further procedure could be performed.

Case 34

A 24-year-old woman presented with repeated episodes of severe anaemia. There was marked pallor with a haemoglobin of 5.6 g/dl and iron deficiency indices of MCV 63 fl and MCH 23.2 pg. Faecal occult bloods were consistently positive. She had no history of menorrhagia and urinalysis was negative. There was no evidence of bruising or lymphadenopathy. No arteriovenous malformations were present within the mouth and the abdomen felt normal. Rectal examination confirmed the presence of positive occult bloods but no frank blood was present. Vaginal examination was normal.

Investigations

Full blood count as above. Clinical chemistry normal. Gastroscopy normal. Barium enema normal. Colonoscopy normal. Barium meal and follow-through normal.

Questions

What is the likely cause for this lady's recurrent anaemia? How should this be investigated and treated?

Discussion

Obscure gastrointestinal bleeding in a young woman is rare. The most likely diagnosis is that of a bleeding Meckel's diverticulum and this is related to the presence of ectopic gastric mucosa within the diverticulum itself. Small bowel tumours such as angiomas, fibromas and leiomyomas may also bleed. In addition, vascular malformations within the gut are associated with gastrointestinal blood loss and Crohn's disease of the small bowel may result in anaemia. In this patient's age group the most common causes of bleeding from the gastrointestinal tract are peptic ulceration, ulcerative colitis and gastrointestinal malignancy which can be excluded by the presence of a normal gastroscopy, colonoscopy, barium enema and barium meal and follow through. Further investigations to ascertain the site of bleeding included small bowel enema. This radiographic technique allows a more detailed visualization of the small bowel mucosa and will often detect small abnormalities and the presence of a Meckel's diverticulum. In addition, chromium-labelled red blood cells can be given intravenously and scans may be taken of the abdomen. The site of bleeding may be seen in selected cases. Angiography is often of value in these patients as arteriovenous malformations, tumour circulation and exact sites of blood loss may be identified. Technetium scans have been advocated for the detection of a Meckel's diverticulum. Technetium is concentrated in peptic cells contained within the ectopic gastric mucosa in these diverticula. Despite early promise, however, these scans are frequently negative, as was the case in this patient, even though a Meckel's diverticulum with gastric mucosa was present.

Meckel's diverticula themselves occur in approximately 2% of the population. They are related to a remnant of the vitellointestinal duct and are situated on the antimesenteric border of the small bowel, about 2 feet from the ileo-caecal valve. In most patients these diverticula remain asymptomatic. When symptomatic, approximately 50% of patients present with bleeding, 25% with obstruction and roughly 25% with inflammation or diverticulitis. Obstruction may be related to volvulus or intussusception. A Meckel's diverticulum is a true diverticulum containing all layers of the intestinal wall; it measures from 1 to 10 cm in length and may contain ectopic tissue of gastric or pancreatic origin.

In this patient with anaemia and persistently positive occult bloods all investigations were normal including small bowel enema, angiography and technetium scan. In such a situation an exploratory laparotomy was indicated.

At laparotomy, a 5 cm Meckel's diverticulum was present and this was subsequently resected. The Meckel's diverticulum was opened and found to contain a small peptic ulcer with ectopic gastric mucosa. Postoperatively she has remained well after follow-up of 2 years.

This case serves to emphasise that despite the plethora of tests available for investigating these patients, frequently the diagnosis is only made at exploratory laparotomy.

Case 35

A 51-year-old man presented with a 6-month history of 2-stone weight loss, lethargy, exhaustion and anorexia. There was neither history of abdominal pain, vomiting, change of bowel habit nor melaena. There was no relevant past medical history and the patient was not on any drug therapy. He was a non-smoker and non-drinker. Examination revealed a tender mass in the right iliac fossa but no other abnormality. His haemoglobin concentration was 8.9 g/dl, white cell count $9.9 \times 10^9/l$, haematocrit 35%, mean corpuscular volume 68 fl, mean corpuscular haemoglobin 21.5 pg and mean corpuscular haemoglobin concentration 31.0 g/dl. The erythrocyte sedimentation rate was 70 mm in the first hour. A blood film showed marked anisocytosis and poikilocytosis. Liver function tests were normal.

Questions

How should the patient be investigated?
What is the appropriate treatment?

Discussion

Faecal occult blood estimations were carried out and were found to be strongly positive on three consecutive occasions. A chest X-ray showed no abnormality. Barium enema showed a large mass with an irregular surface, filling the caecum. The features were those of a caecal carcinoma.

The combination of anorexia, anaemia and asthenia, even in the absence of any direct findings in the abdomen, suggest the presence of malignant disease. Whilst benign conditions, such as pernicious anaemia may produce this symptom complex, these are rare and the possibility of a malignancy must firstly be excluded. The most common malignancies presenting in this way are carcinomas of the caecum, stomach and bronchus. The mass in the right iliac fossa in this patient, together with the positive faecal occult blood estimations, suggest the presence of carcinoma of the caecum; this was subsequently confirmed on barium enema.

At operation, there was a large caecal carcinoma invading through the serosa of the posterior aspect of the caecum into the posterior abdominal wall. Large fleshy lymph nodes were present in the caecal mesentery. The right ureter was adherent to the tumour but not directly invaded. A formal right hemicolectomy was performed, excising approximately 10 cm of terminal ileum and the proximal third of the transverse colon along with the ascending colon and caecum. The mesentery was identified taking care not to damage the second part of the duodenum; all the enlarged nodes visible in the mesentery were removed. An ileo-transverse anastomosis was then performed. Pathological examination of the resected specimen showed a well-differentiated adenocarcinoma of the caecum which was penetrating the full thickness of the bowel wall. Both resection lines were free of tumour, but tumour was present in 3 out of 5 mesenteric lymph nodes examined (Duke's stage C).

The patient made an uneventful postoperative recovery but 1 year later presented with right-sided abdominal pain and further weight loss. The carcino-embryonic antigen concentration which had been less than 5 µg/l during the postoperative follow-up had risen to 27 µg/l. A further laparotomy was performed to reveal the presence of a mass close to the previous ileo-colonic anastomosis. In addition, several loops of small intestine were involved with the mass, but the liver remained clear of tumour. The mass was resected along with 40 cm of small intestine and the patient made an uneventful postoperative recovery. Radiotherapy was considered but deemed inappropriate so the patient was treated with chlorambucil (5 mg/day) and prednisolone (10 mg/day). The patient's condition slowly deteriorated over the next 11 months, the concentration of carcino-embryonic antigen rose steadily to 360 µg/l and the patient died 2 years after his initial resection.

In carcinoma of the caecum, bowel symptoms are often completely absent. Rectal bleeding and the passage of mucus are uncommon; but the patient may present with intestinal obstruction. An abdominal mass, however, is frequently present, and faecal occult blood estimations are usually positive. Nausea and vomiting occur in a small proportion of patients. Obstruction of the appendicular lumen by tumour may give rise to acute appendicitis. The treatment is by right hemicolectomy ensuring that at least 5 cm of apparently normal bowel on each side of the tumour is resected. There is little or no role for either radiotherapy or chemotherapy in the treatment of this condition.

Case 36

A 48-year-old man presented with a 3-month history of increasing constipation with occasional and intermittent bouts of diarrhoea. Two months after the onset of his symptoms he developed pain in the left iliac fossa. A barium enema showed an annular stricture in the proximal sigmoid colon which was 5 cm in length, with shouldering of the proximal and distal extremities. The radiological features were those of a sigmoid colon carcinoma. A chest X-ray showed no abnormality but an ultrasound scan of the liver revealed a large solitary metastasis in the right lobe.

Questions

What is the surgical approach to this problem?
How should the solitary metastasis be approached

Discussion

The initial surgical approach involves resecting the primary tumour and assessing the extent of spread, in particular the extent of the solitary metastasis within the right lobe of the liver. Great care must be taken to ensure, as far as is feasible, that the metastasis is confined to the right lobe of the liver and that there is not widespread lymphatic involvement along the para-aortic chain. At the first operation a sigmoid colectomy with end-to-end primary anastomosis of the colon is performed.

A period of 6 to 8 weeks should then be allowed for recovery from the colectomy; the ultrasound scan should then be repeated and selective coeliac axis angiography carried out. Computerised tomography may also be helpful. Provided that the hepatic metastasis remains confined to the right lobe of the liver, a right hepatic lobectomy may be performed where the liver substance is divided between the right and left surgical lobes. Although the chances of cure are very remote, several cases reported recently have survived for periods in excess of 1 or 2 years following this approach. Left untreated, few with hepatic metastases will survive 1 year.

A further therapeutic option for the patient with hepatic metastases is to use chemotherapy. 5-fluouracil is the drug most commonly employed and may be administered orally, intravenously, or directly into the portal vein following cannulation of the umbilical ligament at operation. Radiotherapy has no proven role in the treatment of hepatic metastases.

Case 37

A 63-year-old man presented with a short history of passage of gas in his urine. For several years prior to the onset of this symptom he had had intermittent bouts of left iliac fossa pain with constipation, interrupted by an occasional bout of diarrhoea. He had also been prone to excess flatulence and abdominal distension. The passage of gas in the urine had developed 2 weeks prior to his presentation and was not associated with urinary frequency, dysuria or haematuria. Nocturia averaged twice nightly. The patient denied the passage of mucus or blood per rectum. Examination revealed tenderness in the left iliac fossa and an easily palpable sigmoid colon. There was a little guarding on the left side of the abdomen, but no abdominal rigidity or rebound tenderness was present. Rectal examination revealed no abnormality.

Questions

How should this patient be investigated?
What is the differential diagnosis?
What treatment is indicated

Discussion

A mid-stream specimen of urine revealed a coliform infection. The haemoglobin was 12.6 g/dl. The white cell count was $12.5 \times 10^9/l$ and ESR 43 mm in the first hour. A rigid sigmoidoscope was passed to 15 cm from the anal verge, and no abnormality was seen on this examination. Flexible sigmoidoscopy was then performed; this showed the characteristic openings of diverticula in the sigmoid colon. The colonic mucosa in the lower sigmoid appeared inflamed and the lumen was narrowed, but no proliferative lesion was seen within the bowel lumen. A plain abdominal X-ray showed no evidence of intestinal obstruction and the gas pattern within the intestine was normal. No gas could be seen in the bladder on this examination. A double-contrast barium enema was then carried out; this showed diverticular disease predominantly affecting the sigmoid colon, but also extending into the descending colon, with a smaller number of diverticula in the transverse and ascending colons. There was some narrowing in the lower sigmoid colon and evidence of muscular spasm, which did not relax during the period in which the barium enema was carried out. A small amount of contrast material was seen to pass from the lower sigmoid colon into the bladder, a narrow track being identified between the two structures.

The presenting symptom here is described as pneumaturia and is due to a colo-vesical fistula. The most common pathological process giving rise to such a fistula is diverticular disease of the colon. It may also occur with colonic malignancies and with Crohn's disease. Ulcerative colitis, ischaemic colitis and the irritable bowel syndrome have not been associated with vesico-colic fistula, but carcinoma of the bladder in the advanced stages may give rise to this problem. Cystoscopy should be carried out to exclude this, but the fistula is frequently invisible on this examination, the only abnormality being a localised patch of cystitis in relation to the site of entry of the fistula into the bladder.

The treatment of this condition is surgical. If the fistula is left, it is unlikely to close spontaneously and there is always the risk of renal damage occurring as a result of persistent severe urinary tract infection and also the possibility of septicaemia. The colon should be prepared with an aperient, such as Picolax, and one or two phosphate enemas should be given. Following the bacteriologist's report of the urine culture, an appropriate broad-spectrum antibiotic which is excreted in the urine should be given, although it is unlikely that this will completely eradicate the infection so long as the fistula persists. At operation, there are usually dense adhesions between the vault of the bladder and the diverticulum which has penetrated the bladder wall. These two structures should be separated, after which a small hole may then be apparent in the bladder. However, this is not always the case and sometimes following separation the site of penetration of the bladder is not apparent. If a substantial hole exists in the bladder wall the margins of this should be excised and the bladder repaired with 2 or 3 layers of catgut suture material. Having separated the colon from the bladder, a sigmoid colectomy or, in the case of more extensive diverticular disease, a more radical colonic resection should be performed. An end-to-end anastomosis of the colon may be carried out provided that the colonic preparation has been adequate, and that there was no obstruction of the colon at the time of surgery; otherwise a temporary loop transverse colostomy should be performed. This minimizes the risk of further fistula formation between the suture line on the colon and the site at which the bladder has been closed. The temporary colostomy may be closed 1 month after the operation when the patient's clinical condition is satisfactory and when the colonic anastomosis has been demonstrated to be intact. A further technical consideration which the surgeon should take advantage of, if possible, is the interposition of omentum between the colonic anastomosis and the site of bladder closure.

Diverticula of the colon are hernias or out-pouchings of the mucosa through defects in the colonic musculature. The defects coincide with sites at which blood vessels penetrate the colonic wall. In Western countries the disease is extremely common, affecting over one third of people over the age of 60 years. However, in Africa and the greater part of South East Asia it is rare; this has been attributed to the taking of a high residue diet in these latter areas. Females are more commonly affected than males, and people of African or Asian extraction living in westernized countries for long periods of time and eating westernized diets develop approximately the same incidence of the disease as the indigenous Caucasians.

Hypertrophy of both the longitudinal and circular muscle predominantly in the sigmoid colon gives rise to increased intra-colonic pressure which predisposes to the herniation of the mucosa throught sites of weakness in the colonic wall. This situation is exacerbated by taking a low residue diet. The fundamental pathological lesion of muscular hypertrophy is present in the longitudinal muscle as well as the circular, and in 75% of cases the disease is confined to the sigmoid colon. Acute inflammation around the diverticulum is referred to as diverticulitis and dense adhesions can then form between this inflamed diverticulum and adjacent structures, such as the bladder. Fistula formation can occur as a result of such an attack of acute diverticulitis. Other complications of diverticular disease are colonic bleeding and abscess formation. Since diverticular disease is so common, the surgeon must avoid overlooking a colonic neoplasm within an area of diverticular disease. Whilst there is no evidence that diverticular disease predisposes to colonic cancer, the two conditions are frequently seen to concur. A fistula may also develop between the colon and the vagina, or between the colon and the abdominal wall; however, the latter is less common in diverticular disease than it is in Crohn's disease. Uncomplicated diverticular disease should be treated conservatively with a high-residue diet and bran supplementation, together with an anti-spasmodic, such as mebeverine. Where medical treatment fails in the uncomplicated situation, surgery must be considered, the most commonly performed operation being sigmoidcolectomy but sigmoid myotomy, division of the circular muscle along the length of the sigmoid colon, has been advocated and shown to be effective, at least in short term management. Where abscess or colonic perforation has occurred, emergency surgery is indicated. Following haemorrhage from diverticular disease emergency surgery is rarely required, since bleeding most commonly spontaneously arrests. The mortality of the disease is low, but prolonged morbidity is considerable; approximately 25% of patients develop peridiverticular inflammation within a 10-year period and free perforation occurs in approximately 5%. It is possible that the awareness within the community of the benefits of high-residue diets has reduced the number of complications arising from diverticular disease of the colon.

Case 38

A man of 88 years of age who lived alone and had recently become confused was admitted as an emergency. The patient who had lost his wife 16 years earlier, lived in a flat in a deprived inner city area. He had been found lying on the floor of his flat in a dehydrated state by a neighbour. His only complaints were of vague abdominal pain.

He was unclean and unshaven with gross bilateral leg oedema and chronic venous insufficiency with ulceration. His abdomen was moderately distended and tympanitic, peristalsis was also visible. Bowel sounds were high-pitched and somewhat fatigued. Rectal examination was normal.

Questions

How should the patient be investigated?
What treatment is appropriate?

Discussion

The initial management of the patient involves full clinical assessment, particularly of his circulatory state, and then resuscitation. The patient was quite grossly dehydrated and this was corrected by the infusion of crystalloids. An erect and supine plain abdominal X-ray showed gross colonic dilatation, the transverse diameter of the colon being 20 cm at its widest part. From the X-ray it was not possible to identify which part of the bowel was so dilated, as the whole of the abdominal cavity seemed to be filled by this grossly-dilated loop. It was assumed that the features were those of a sigmoid volvulus, but the possibility of a caecal volvulus needed to be excluded.

The most common form of colonic volvulus, sigmoid volvulus, is particularly liable to occur in those elderly individuals in whom there is a long history of chronic constipation and in whom a long sigmoid loop is suspended from a long mesentery on a short base. These patients are often socially deprived, perhaps mentally retarded and are frequently found in long-term care institutions. The features of intestinal obstruction are often absent until late in the acute exacerbation of the disorder. Abdominal distension becomes manifest and colicky lower abdominal pain is also a feature. Complete constipation gradually develops with absence of the passage of bowel gas. Borborygmi occur as the abdomen becomes progressively distended and vomiting accrues late in the course of the disorder. Gross abdominal distension develops and peristalsis is visible. Plain abdominal X-ray usually reveals a grossly-dilated sigmoid colon which often fills the whole of the left side of the abdomen up to the diaphragm. The more proximal colon becomes distended and fluid levels are commonly seen in the small bowel.

Conservative treatment should be employed firstly. It may be possible to untwist the volvulus by the passage of a large rubber rectal tube which is inserted through a sigmoidoscope into the bowel lumen at the site of the apex of the volvulus. Gaseous decompression is classically impressive. The flexible colonoscope has also been used to decompress the bowel.

Frequently adequate decompression by this route fails and, in addition, if strangulation of the bowel is suspected on clinical grounds, laparotomy is required. The volvulus should be untwisted and the sigmoid colon then resected, after which an end colostomy is formed. The bowel can be reanastomosed at a later date providing the patient's general condition permits this.

Case 39

A 43-year-old woman gave an 18-year history of diarrhoea with the passage of mucus and blood per rectum. A diagnosis of ulcerative colitis had been made in the early clinical stages of the disease and the patient had been treated with salazopyrin, in doses up to 2 g daily, and prednisolone. The former drug had been used throughout most of the course of the disease but the patient had become intolerant of it in later years, and the dose had had to be reduced. The latter drug had been used topically in the exacerbations of the disease. Fifteen years after first developing the disease, the patient underwent hysterectomy for menorrhagia following which her bowel disease was exacerbated, with the patient passing up to 20 bowel actions daily over the subsequent years. This more debilitating phase of the disease had responded poorly to medication. There had been no skin, eye or joint problems.

Barium enema, which had been performed on 5 occasions during the course of the disease, showed a total colitis with marked narrowing of the rectum and colon, loss of haustra and an increase in the presacral space. Colonoscopy revealed a total colitis with severe ulceration, pseudopolyposis and areas denuded of the rectal mucosa. Multiple biopsies were taken. The patient was mildly anaemic (11.6 g/dl), serum electrolytes and liver function were normal.

Questions

What are the indications for surgical treatment in ulcerative colitis?
What operative treatment should be offered?

Discussion

This woman clearly suffered from the severe manifestations of ulcerative colitis which was beginning to produce chronic ill-health and social dislocation. The condition has a prevalence of 40 to 80 cases per 100 000 population in Britain and a mortality of 0.5 to 0.7 per 100 000 per annum.

The absolute indications for emergency surgical treatment are colonic perforation, massive haemorrhage, progressive colonic dilation and failure to respond to intravenous steroids, fluid replacement and bed rest. Early elective surgical treatment is required for proven malignant change in the colon or rectum or nodular lesions with high-grade cellular dysplasia. None of these factors were present in this case but, in addition to the chronic ill-health and failure to respond to medical treatment, the patient was entering the high-risk stage of the disease as regards malignant damage. The colonoscopic biopsies had not shown malignant change but, after 20 years of active disease, patients with total colonic involvement run a high-risk of developing carcinoma which can occur at a relatively early age. The incidence of carcinoma rises to approximately 25% after 25 years of active disease; the majority of patients developing cancer having total or subtotal colitis.

The choice of elective operation ranges between panproctocolectomy and ileostomy; colectomy with ileostomy and either subsequent excision of the rectum or ileo-rectal anastomosis; colectomy with immediate ileo-rectal anastomosis; and colectomy, mucosal proctectomy, ileal reservoir formation and ileo-anal anastomosis.

Panproctocolectomy with ileostomy has the advantage of being curative, with a low mortality and morbidity. Convalescence is shortest following this procedure though perineal problems such as delayed healing and persistent sinus formation can occur. The Brooke's ileostomy is simple to create and usually trouble-free. Conversely, ileorectal anastomosis, either immediate or delayed, is a controversial method of treatment. Despite the advantage of retaining continence the operation, by preserving the rectum, leaves the most diseased portion of the bowel intact. Thus diarrhoea continues, often with tenesmus, bleeding and mucus. There is a risk of malignant change in the rectal stump and sometimes the non-gastrointestinal manifestations of the disease either flare up or fail to resolve. Even when this form of therapy is confined to the patient with only moderate rectal disease and a distensible rectum, approximately one third to one half eventually have to undergo rectal excision.

Mucosal proctectomy, ileal reservoir formation and ileo-anal anastomosis is probaly the ideal operation. In particular, it preserves continence, removes the whole of the disease and should have a low incidence of subsequent sexual dysfunction. The colon and upper rectum are completely excised. The mid-rectum is divided and the mucosa is stripped off the rectal remnant. Ulcerative colitis, being a disease of the mucosa, is thus completely cured; however, it is of paramount importance that none of the rectal mucosa is left behind as this could subsequently undergo malignant change. The ileal pouch can be formed in one of two ways. The Parks 'S' pouch consists of a reservoir constructed from three adjacent 15 cm loops of terminal ileum anastomosed together with a short efferent loop; this is then anastomosed to the ano-rectal junction. The 'J' pouch consists of two adjacent 15 cm loops of ileum anastomosed together before the apex of the 'J' is anastomosed to the ano-rectal junction. A temporary loop ileostomy is required with each of these pouches and this is retained for about 3 months. This more extensive surgical treatment is still undergoing evaluation.

It is the author's practice to describe in detail the operations of panproctocolectomy with ileostomy and mucosal proctectomy to the patients, indicating their advantages and disadvantages before discussing the patient's attitude to these forms of treatment. Usually, the patient is keen to have a mucosal proctectomy and retain continence.

For the patient with an ileostomy who is concerned about retaining continence an ileal reservoir, as described by Kock, can be created and fixed behind the anterior abdominal wall. The reservoir is created by anastomosing three loops of ileum and is made continent by the retrograde intussusception of the terminal ileum just distal to the reservoir. The stoma is small, lies flush with the skin, can be low on the abdominal wall and no appliance is necessary. Evacuation is achieved by passing a catheter through the valve into the reservoir.

Case 40

A 74-year-old woman presented with an episode of heavy, fresh rectal bleeding. The episode had occurred spontaneously and dramatically, there having been no associated and no predisposing symptoms. On two previous occasions the patient had witnessed similar but smaller bleeding episodes. At the time of admission to hospital the patient was in a mild state of shock which rapidly and spontaneously corrected itself. She had an aortic systolic murmur, but otherwise no abnormality was found on clinical examination. Following the previous episode of bleeding, a barium enema had been performed which showed diverticular disease of the sigmoid colon, the rest of the examination was normal. Sigmoidoscopy was normal, there were no haemorrhoids present.

Questions

What is the differential diagnosis?
How should this patient be investigated?
What form of management is appropriate?

Discussion

This clinical situation presents one of the most difficult problems in colo-rectal surgery. The differential diagnosis rests chiefly between angiodysplasia of the colon and bleeding from diverticular disease. In the differential diagnosis the exclusion of massive upper gastrointestinal tract bleeding from, particularly, either a duodenal ulcer or oesophageal varices is mandatory. Other conditions lower down the gut which may require to be excluded are bleeding from a Meckel's diverticulum, from Crohn's disease, ulcerative colitis or angiomatous malformations of the colon.

After excluding, or dealing with massive blood loss by transfusion, the most pertinent investigations are colonoscopy and selective angiography. Gastroduodenoscopy should be performed.

Colonoscopy under these circumstances may be difficult and is often unhelpful. If the bleeding is continuing, blood rapidly becomes dispersed throughout the colon and lies within the diverticula in the sigmoid. The examination is complicated since the field of view tends to be obscured by blood which may be impossible to aspirate through the endoscope. Unless fresh blood is actively emerging from a diverticulum, this disorder cannot be implicated as the cause of haemorrhage. If haemorrhage has stopped and the bowel has been adequately prepared, the endoscopist may see the classical submucosal arteriovenous malformations of angiodysplasia transilluminated through the mucosa. These may be present anywhere in the colon, or occasionally more proximally, but usually they arise in the caecum. The endoscopist may only rarely be able to identify the site of haemorrhage in the colon.

Selective arteriography is the most useful investigation in diagnosing angiodysplasia. Both superior and inferior mesenteric cannulations may show the classical features of arteriovenous malformations with venous lakes within the submucosa. Where bleeding is active and greater than 1ml/min the contrast may pool in the gut lumen. Isotopic studies using radiolabelled red blood cells (or occasionally white cells) may be helpful by demonstrating a 'blush' of increased radioactivity in the region of the site of bleeding.

Frequently these investigations are negative and treatment must be decided upon clinical grounds. Angiodysplasia is statistically the most likely cause of this patient's bleeding and is most likely to be affecting the right rather than the left side of the colon. Conversely, the patient could be bleeding from her left-sided diverticular disease or the angiodysplasia could be affecting the left side of the colon. Continued bleeding or another bleeding episode is very likely to occur.

The choice of surgical treatment results between right hemicolectomy, left hemicolectomy or total colectomy with ileo-rectal anastomosis. The rationale for right hemicolectomy is that the right side of the colon bears the brunt of bleeding from angiodysplasia. Left hemicolectomy, or sigmoid colectomy should only be performed if the surgeon has good evidence that the diverticular disease is the source of bleeding. Total colectomy is most likely to be curative by excising most potential sites of bleeding from angiodysplasia and eradicating the diverticula. Against this is the more extensive nature of the surgery and the inevitable diarrhoea which will develop postoperatively. A further clinical factor which is suggestive of angiodysplasia in this case is the finding of aortic stenosis, the two conditions are connected.

A total colectomy with ileo-rectal anastomosis was performed with a good clinical result and the patient has remained well without further bleeding. Histological examination of the resected specimen showed the features of angiodysplasia in the caecum.

Case 41

A 68-year-old man presented with a 6-week history of fresh rectal bleeding, increased frequency of defaecation and a sensation of incomplete evacuation of the rectum. The blood loss occurred predominantly with defaecation and was small in volume usually surrounding the surface of the motion. When flatus was passed small amounts of blood and a little mucus were present, and the stool had become coated in mucus. There had been no heavy bleeding. The patient denied frank diarrhoea, but had developed an increased frequency of bowel habit. He denied any abdominal or perineal pain, and there was no history of abdominal distension. Digital examination of the rectum revealed a tumour with its lower palpable extremity 8 cm from the anal verge. This extended proximally beyond the tip of the examining finger and appeared to be involving just less than half the rectal circumference at its widest point. The tumour was firm and appeared to be mobile. Sigmoidoscopy revealed an ulcerating carcinoma, extending from 8 to 13 cm from the anal verge; the lesion had a central area of ulceration with raised edges and felt firm on biopsy performed through the sigmoidoscope. Chest X-ray showed no abnormality; biochemical tests of liver function and an ultrasound scan of the liver were within normal limits. Barium enema demonstrated the lesion in the rectum but showed no evidence of a metachronous tumour in the more proximal colon. Histological examination of the biopsy specimen revealed adenocarcinoma of the rectum. Carcino-embryonic antigen (CEA) was estimated to be at baseline levels.

Questions

Which factors affect prognosis?
What is the appropriate treatment of this condition?

Discussion

The two factors which affect the prognosis of carcinoma of the rectum are the surgical staging of the tumour and its histological grade. The method of surgical staging employed is that first described by Dukes in 1932, which is as follows: Dukes grade A describes spread into the submucosa or muscle of the bowel but not beyond, with no lymph node involvement. Dukes grade B indicates spread beyond the muscle coat into the pericolic or perirectal tissue, but without lymph node involvement. In Dukes grade C1, lymph nodes are involved in close proximity to the tumour and in C2, more distant lymphatic spread. Although Dukes did not originally describe a grade D, this is sometimes used to describe the patient in whom there are distant blood-borne metastases to, for example, the liver. Dukes grade A lesions have an excellent 5-year survival of over 90%, Dukes B lesions 5-year survival of some 65% and in Dukes C lesions the 5-year survival is approximately 25%. Regrettably, a high proportion of tumours are Dukes grade C at the time of presentation.

The histological grade of the tumour is determined by (i) the degree of tubule formation, (ii) variability in size, shape and staining of nuclei, (iii) the number of mitotic figures and (iv) the arrangements of cells and nuclei within the tubules. Well-differentiated tumours have a much better 5-year survival rate than those which are poorly differentiated. The surgical treatment of carcinoma of the middle rectum remains controversial; the two options being anterior resection of the rectum with an end-to-end colorectal anastomosis or abdominoperineal resection. Anterior resection has the obvious aesthetic advantage of the maintenence of an intact gastrointestinal tract with normal sphincter function and thus complete continence. Abdominoperineal resection of the rectum, whilst perhaps being a more radical cancer operation, has the disadvantage of providing the patient with a permanent end colostomy and additional complications which might accrue are impotence and bladder dysfunction. A factor which must be considered in deciding upon the most appropriate form of surgical treatment is the extent of intramucosal and submucosal spread from the macroscopically obvious limit of the tumour. Spread in a distal direction is usually confined to a distance of 1 cm and rarely extends beyond 2 cm from the visible lower limit of the tumour. Thus, in this case, where the tumour has its lower edge 8 cm from the anal verge, the surgeon must consider making his site of resection at 6 cm from the anal verge in order to be sure of clearing the tumour. The feasibility of such a level of resection depends upon the size of the patient, the degree of local invasion related to the tumour, and the extent of lymphatic involvement. Whilst it is technically feasible to carry out anterior restorative resection for tumours situated at this level, there is a higher incidence of local recurrence, and some surgeons take the precaution of swabbing the lumen of the rectum with a 1 in 500 solution of mercuric perchloride; this must not be allowed to spill into the peritoneal cavity. In recent years, there has been a greater tendency for surgeons to carry out low anterior resection using intraluminal stapling. The decision of whether to use a stapling gun or a hand-sutured anastomosis largely depends upon the experience and preference of the individual surgeon. For low stapled anterior resection, a purse-string suture has to be placed around the edge of the divided rectum, and the technical difficulty which might be encountered in inserting this purse-string may be similar to that in performing a hand-sutured anastomosis. The author prefers to suture the anastomosis by hand. Inserting the purse-string into the proximal bowel can easily be carried out using a special serrated device. In this clinical situation the decision whether or not to perform an anterior resection must often be made by the surgeon at the time of laparotomy. If there is any doubt that adequate clearance cannot be obtained in performing a restorative resection, then the surgeon should carry out abdominoperineal resection of the rectum. Occasionally, despite full mobilisation of the rectum to the level of the anal canal, it may be difficult to insert a purse-string suture into the distal bowel. Under these circumstances, the rectum is divided 1 to 2 cm above the anorectal ring and from the perineal aspect the surgeon can suture the anorectal stump employing a transanal approach. A Park's anal retractor is useful in facilitating this surgical technique. Having achieved the lower purse-string, a colo-anal anastomosis can then be carried out using the staple gun. As an alternative to this, for the very low anterior section, some surgeons (e.g. Turnbull, Cutait and Hughes) have described a pull-through technique with an external anastomosis.

The question of whether or not to perform adjuvant radiotherapy has recently been investigated in several clinical studies. Whilst it has been claimed that preoperative radiotherapy can convert tumours of an advanced Duke's stage to a less advanced stage, the overall evidence has shown no difference in survival or in rates of local recurrence and distant metastases following the use of adjuvant radiotherapy. There is little place for chemotherapy in the treatment of advanced rectal cancer but adjuvant chemotherapy administered into the portal vein in the immediate postoperative period may confer some slight reduction in the incidence of hepatic metastases.

The overall postoperative mortality for curative resection of carcinoma of the rectum is of the order of 5%. The ultimate 5-year survival depends upon the Duke's grade and the differentiation of the tumour, as has already been stated.

For advanced tumours which are fixed and unresectable, an end colostomy should be performed employing a Hartmann's procedure. Where hepatic metastases are present but where the tumour is resectable, resection should be performed to overcome the local problems associated with the tumour. Regrettably, the overall survival from carcinoma of the rectum has not improved in the last 30 years, despite technical innovations and the increased understanding of tumour behaviour.

Case 42

A 32-year-old man presented with a history of continual discharge from the perianal region. This discharge comprised of a mixture of mucus and pus, with occasional episodes of bleeding. His bowels functioned normally. There had been no history of weight loss and his appetite was good. In the previous 3 years, he had undergone 2 operations for incision and drainage of an ischiorectal abscess. No abnormality could be detected in the abdomen. External examination of the rectum revealed a perineal opening of a probable fistula on the left side of the anus postero-laterally (signified clinically at 4 o'clock), approximately 3 cm from the anal verge. Internal rectal examination suggested an internal opening in the same position. Sigmoidoscopy showed no evidence of colitis or mucosal abnormalities within the rectum. All blood tests were normal.

Questions

Discuss the pathology of perianal fistula.
How should this be managed surgically?

Discussion

The most common cause of perianal fistula is as a sequel to an abscess in the perianal region. This may be the result of spontaneous drainage, or inadequate surgical drainage. Perianal fistulae are also commonly seen as a complication of Crohn's Disease, especially where the large bowel is involved in that condition. Tuberculosis, carcinoma of the rectum and trauma are infrequent causes of perianal fistula. Perianal fistula as a sequel to an abscess is resultant on infection starting in an anal gland and the fistulous tract is lined by granulation tissue and may contain pus. The walls themselves are composed of dense fibrous tissue which can often be felt through the skin. Fistulae have both an internal and an external opening, communicating between two epithelial surfaces. Most fistulae are low lying below the levator ani muscle and only rarely are high fistulae seen. Fistulas have been classified as most commonly intersphincteric (70% of fistula) and these are related to infection in the anal gland which lies in the intersphincteric plane. In these fistulae, the internal opening is in the rectum and the fistulous tract passes through the internal sphincter and out into the perianal region. Occasionally side tracts are also present and these may pass upwards into the rectal wall. Transphincteric fistulae account for approximately 25% of all perianal fistulae and these tracts pass through both the internal and external sphincters. If the tract passes through the lower part of the muscles of the sphincters then these are more easily treated. If the tract passes through the upper part of the sphincter mass, then these are extremely difficult to treat, as incontinence may supervene. Suprasphincteric fistulae account for approximately 4 to 5% of all cases and in these the tract passes through the puborectalis above all the muscles responsible for continence. Extra sphincteric fistulae (1% of all fistulae) are the least common of perianal fistulae. These pass from the rectum directly to the skin through the muscles although they may have a side extension to the anal gland. Although fistulae are frequently simple, occasionally the tracts can have wide ramifications with horse shoe tract formation and multiple external openings. This is particularly the case with Crohn's Disease where the fistulae tend not to follow the anatomical planes, as do fistulae following simple abscess formation.

Perianal abscesses should always be treated promptly. Careful examination at the time of drainage should reveal an internal opening and if this is present the abscess must be carefully drained and the entire tract laid open. Bacteriological swabs taken at this stage are helpful as faecal organisms are within the abscess if a fistulous tract is present. The presence of non faecal organisms (e.g. *Staphylococcus aureus*) within the abscess suggests that there is no true fistula present. Once the presence of a fistula has been determined the method of treatment is to open the fistulous tract to secure free drainage and to allow the tract to heal from its base. If the fistula is intersphincteric, or a low transphincteric fistula, surgery can be easily performed by placing a probe through it, being careful not to create false passages, and then by opening directly onto this. The fistulous tract should then be curetted and all unhealthy granulation tissue removed. Careful postoperative dressing will allow rapid healing. A specimen of the fistulous tract should be removed for pathological examination to exclude the presence of perianal Crohn's disease. High transphincteric, suprasphincteric and extra sphincteric fistulas are difficult to manage and are probably best treated in specialised unit. Extreme care must be taken to prevent the patient from becoming incontinent as a result of sphincter damage. Frequently a staged procedure is needed and a defunctioning transverse colostomy may be also required to permit full healing to occur. Seton sutures are also occasionally used where there are difficult high fistulae to allow free drainage during surgical treatment. These sutures allow a staged procedure to be performed without interfering with anal continence. In general the prognosis of patients with difficult fistulae is not good, since fistulae often recur, some patients become incontinent and often a severely deformed anus results. Additionally the wounds may take a long time to heal.

The present patient was given a disposable enema prior to surgery. At operation, carried out in the lithotomy position, a probe was passed from the external to internal opening. Examination revealed an intersphincteric fistula. A knife was used to cut down onto the probe and the whole fistulous tract demonstrated. The walls of the tract were removed and curetted and pathological examination of the excised tissue showed no evidence of Crohn's disease. Postoperatively he underwent daily dressings with salt baths and within 3 weeks the wound had healed completely with maintenance of full continence. At 3-year follow-up he had no further problems.

Case 43

A 56-year-old woman presented with a 5-year history of faecal incontinence, sometimes associated with the passage of mucus and small amounts of blood. Her problem had severe social and professional consequences leading her to become very withdrawn, and to follow a solitary existence. She stated that she was not always aware of the passage of faecal material but that in between times defaecation was normal. The stool was normal in consistency and she had neither previous gastrointestinal disorders nor gastrointestinal surgery. There was no history of backache or of injury to her spine. She had three children, all delivered vaginally, without any apparent problems.

On examination of her abdomen there was no abnormality. Anorectal examination revealed obvious soiling of the perianal area but no evidence of previous sphincteric damage, infection or disease. Digital examination excluded neoplasia and revealed a very lax sphincter tone, which the patient had difficulty in voluntarily contracting. Sigmoidoscopy was normal and at this examination there was no evidence of complete rectal prolapse, although second-degree haemorrhoids were present.

Questions

What is the aetiology of anorectal incontinence.
How might the patient be investigated and what is the treatment of choice?

Discussion

Initially the presence of other colo-rectal disorders (e.g. inflammatory bowel disease, faecal impaction with spurious diarrhoea and the irritable bowel syndrome) should be excluded. It is also important to carry out a full neurological examination, testing for evidence of neurological impairment in the lower limbs and sensory abnormalities, particularly in the perianal area. Radiological examination for spinal stenosis or spondylolisthesis should also be performed. The innervation of the levator ani and external sphincter mechanism is from the second, third and fourth sacral segments, via the pudendal nerve. Cord lesions result in spastic paralysis of the sphincter mechanism and cauda aquina lesions in a flaccid paralysis. Impaired sphincter control in both these situations may result in leakage from the anal canal. Peripheral nerve injury to the pudendal nerve may also result in anorectal incontinence. This is probably due to a stretch injury of the pudendal nerve as a result of rectal and perineal descent; injury may also have occurred at childbirth. Abnormal perineal descent may result from repeated straining at stool or rectal prolapse. Entrapment of the nerve beneath the sacro-tuberous ligament may occur.

The patient had second-degree haemorrhoids; these may lead to small amounts of soiling but not to frank incontinence. Muscular disorders (e.g. scleroderma and dermatomyositis) may result in a functional abnormality of the sphincter, and patients with disseminated sclerosis or motor neurone disease may develop incontinence, often as a result of spurious diarrhoea secondary to faecal impaction. Patients who have chronically abused laxatives for many years may, by virtue of the sporadic and induced nature of the bowel action, develop incontinence. In addition, any patient with diarrhoea which is precipitate in its nature as in, for example, post-vagotomy diarrhoea, may be incontinent.

Previous surgical treatment of ano-rectal conditions such as fistula-in-ano and haemorrhoids may also result in incontinence. If fistulae which track above the sphincter mechanism are laid open, permanent sphincter damage may occur. In addition, incontinence has been recorded after excessive stretching of the anorectal musculature in the performance of the Lord's procedure for treating third-degree haemorrhoids.

Clinical evaluation is fundamental, not only to determine the presence of other colo-rectal disorders but also the tone of the sphincter and the patient's voluntary control can be assessed digitally. Rectal prolapse can be excluded by the examining clinician who should attempt to produce prolapse by applying traction to the lower rectal mucosa. The patient may be reluctant to inform the clinician of the prolapse or may not be aware that this is occurring. Electromyographic studies of pudendal nerve function have been carried out, but remain largely a research tool. Manometric studies may show a low resting pressure in the anal canal but are usually unhelpful. A defaecating proctogram may be helpful in assessing perineal descent which is commonly associated with incontinence.

The treatment of anorectal incontinence depends upon the cause; thus every attempt must be made to define accurately the underlying nature of the patient's problem. Simple conditions such as haemorrhoids, which may be contributing to the patient's problem, should be treated promptly and the effect of this therapy on the underlying incontinence should be assessed before more extensive methods of surgery are carried out. When sphincter denervation is thought to result from lower motor neurone lesion or when there is loss of the normal ano-rectal angle as a result of abnormal perineal descent, and when the incontinence is idiopathic, a post-anal repair of the sphincter mechanism, as described by Parks, is the most appropriate form of treatment. The principle of the operation is to create a sharper anorectal angle. The approach is through the perineum and behind the sphincters until the fascia of Waldeyer is reached; this is then divided to allow the posterior rectal wall to be swept forwards. The levator ani muscles are then firmly sutured together and the pubococcygeus and puborectalis muscles are apposed bilaterally by sutures. The external sphincter complex may also be reinforced by sutures. The performance of an apparently adequate Parks post-anal repair is not always successful in curing the patient's incontinence.

Where direct sphincter damage has occurred, reconstruction of the sphincters may be carried out, together with a defunctioning colostomy. When the repair has fully healed and been shown to be adequate, the colostomy may be closed. Elderly, debilitated patients in institutions may develop incontinence; this leads to serious nursing problems, and where the general condition of the patient precludes general anaesthesia and relatively major surgery, a Thiersch wire can be inserted using local anaesthesia.

In patients whose incontinence results from rectal prolapse, this should be assessed and treated in its own right. The incontinence will usually resolve, but if not then a Parks post-anal repair should be performed in addition.

Case 44

A 49-year-old woman presented with a 3-week history of the awareness of a lump in her left breast. She had neither pain in the breast, discharge from the nipple, nor previous history of breast disease. The menarche occurred at the age of 14 years and the patient was pre-menopausal. A maternal aunt had died of breast cancer. The patient was married with a 14-year-old child, whom she had not breast fed. Examination revealed a hard 3 cm diameter lesion in the axillary tail of the breast. There was a minor degree of skin tethering over-lying the centre of the lesion, but no deep fixation, the tumour being completely mobile. In the left axilla a small, relatively soft, mobile lymph node was present, the nature of which was difficult to determine on clinical grounds alone.

Questions

How should the patient be investigated?
What is the treatment of choice?

Discussion

The clinical findings suggest a stage I or possibly stage II carcinoma of the breast. The hard consistency of the tumour and the presence of minor overlying skin tethering are highly suggestive of malignancy. The size of the tumour and absence of deep fixation are in keeping with a stage I neo-plasm. If, however, the palpable node in the left axilla was involved with tumour this mobile node would indicate that the lesion has progressed to stage II. Clinical assessment of axillary lymph nodes can be extremely difficult and there is considerable observer variation. Whether the tumour belongs to stage I or stage II breast cancer would not affect the clinical management; if the tumour were of stage III or IV however, this would materially affect the approach to subse-quent treatment.

The investigation of this patient must be aimed at: (i) con-firming the diagnosis and (ii) accurately assessing the extent of tumour spread.

The 3 commonly used approaches to establish the diag-nosis are Trucut needle biopsy, aspiration cytology and exci-sion biopsy. Trucut needle biopsy and aspiration cytology can be carried out at the time of consultation using a local anaesthetic and thus provide an early diagnosis. The tech-nique is safe but may be subject to a tissue sampling error as a result of which the diagnosis of malignancy may be overlooked. Haematoma formation is the only early complication; there is also a theoretical possibility that tumour cells may be spread either along the track of the needle or into the blood stream. Some surgeons, instead of obtaining a core of tissue with a Trucut needle, perform fine needle aspiration cytology. This, when reported as positive by an experienced cytologist, is a reliable result; however, a negative report should be further investigated.

Excision biopsy may be performed either before, on a separate occasion from any subsequent treatment, or under the same anaesthetic. Whilst the latter method would appear to have the advantage of expediency, it relies on the assessment of a frozen section which may be less accurate than paraffin section. It also has the disadvantage that, psychologically, the patient has to be prepared for mastectomy for what may be a benign lesion requiring only local excision. The excised tumour should be submitted for the assessment of oestrogen (and possibly progesterone) receptor activity which may affect treatment at a later date.

It is important in the initial assessment of the patient to determine, as accurately as is possible, the extent of spread of the tumour. To this end chest X-ray is mandatory; in addition, an isotope bone scan should be carried out. The latter is a more sensitive indicator of bony metastases than radiology. The value of mammography in a patient with an established palpable tumour is not very great but there are those who argue that it may be valuable in detecting early tumours in the opposite breast. Imaging techniques in the assessment of axillary lymph nodes are not very valuable, lymphoscintigraphy has been used but is probably not very accurate. Ultrasound and computerised tomography (CT) have been used in the initial assessment but probably have no established role. These imaging modalities may be valuable in the detection of liver metastases in more advanced disease.

The treatment of early (stages I and II) breast cancer remains controversial. Numerous trials have been reported comparing different surgical approaches with or without radiotherapy. The surgical options are simple mastectomy, radical mastectomy, or modified radical mastectomy. Radiotherapy has been given as a primary treatment to the tumour and, alternatively, as an adjunct to surgery. Most of the studies reported have failed to show a significant difference in long-term survival between simple and radical mastectomy. Similarly, the addition of radiotherapy to surgery does not affect survival but does reduce the incidence of local tumour recurrence. Most surgeons would remove the breast completely, as removal of the lump alone is associated with a high incidence of local recurrence within the same breast, however lumpectomy and radiotherapy is being reassessed and is gaining popularity in some centres.

Attitudes differ regarding the approach to the axilla. Some leave this untouched, arguing that the nodes form a natural defence to the spread of tumour; they may extend this argument even to those with obviously involved lymph nodes. Sampling of the pectoral nodes at the entrance to the axilla has been used by some as an index of disease spread and gives an accurate estimate in about 90 per cent of cases. Those with involved nodes may then be treated by radiotherapy. Other surgeons routinely remove all detectable axillary lymph nodes by block dissection. In the Patey modified radical mastectomy the pectoralis major muscle is preserved, but pectoralis minor is removed along with the axillary nodes.

The authors would suggest that a suitable surgical approach to this patient would be simple mastectomy combined with axillary clearance. We would withhold radiotherapy until local tumour recurrence developed. Some would argue in favour of ovarian irradiation or oophorectomy which seems to delay the onset of recurrent disease by approximately 2 years. Other forms of treatment should be reserved in case of tumour recurrence.

The patient could be offered breast reconstruction in the form of a subpectoral silicone implant, a latissimus dorsi flap, or a combination of both of these techniques. However, patients', and surgeons', attitudes towards such reconstructive techniques vary widely.

Case 45

A 64-year-old woman presented with breathlessness and stated that she had been aware of a lump in her left breast for about 8 months. Whilst painless the lump had increased in size distorting the shape of the breast. In addition, she complained of some pain in the region of the thoracic spine. There was no previous history of breast disease, no nipple discharge and no family history of breast disease. The patient was unmarried with no pregnancies. Examination revealed a fixed tumour in the upper outer quadrant of the left breast with attachment both to the overlying skin and the pectoral muscle. There was a mass of lymph nodes in the axilla which appeared fixed. No nodes could be palpated in either supraclavicular fossa. Examination of the chest revealed an impaired percussion note at the right base with absent breath sounds and impaired vocal resonance and fremitus over that area. Chest X-ray confirmed the presence of a right-sided pleural effusion, and an isotope bone scan showed areas of increased radioactivity in the region of the thoracic spine. An ultrasound scan of the liver showed no evidence of metastases.

Questions

What treatment is appropriate for this patient?

Discussion

The factors to be taken into consideration here are the age of the patient, the nature and the extent of the tumour. Although the patient was 64 years of age she had no other evidence of disease which was likely to reduce her life expectancy apart from the breast cancer. In determining the nature of the tumour both the oestrogen (and possibly progesterone) receptor status of the patient and the degree of histological differentiation may be valuable. The tumour was clearly very extensive, stage IV, with blood spread, bony metastases and a malignant pleural effusion being present.

Curative treatment is out of the question and the decision rests with the most appropriate form of palliation. The upper outer quadrant of the breast including the tumour, should be excised and the tissue submitted for assessment of oestrogen receptor activity. Oestrogen-receptor positive tumours are thought to be more likely to respond to hormonal manipulative therapy than receptor negative tumours.

There is a degree of correlation between the cellular differentation of a tumour and its receptor activity, well-differentiated tumours being more likely to contain oestrogen receptors and therefore to respond well.

The forms of hormonal manipulative therapy available to the postmenopausal woman with advanced breast cancer are: (i) the antio-estrogen tamoxifen, (ii) hypophysectomy or (iii) adrenalectomy, the latter two effects may be achieved chemically rather than surgically by the drug aminoglutethimide. Tamoxifen is an extremely safe drug with a minimum of side-effects. It achieves its anti-oestrogen effect in an oral dose of 10 mg 3 times daily. Once introduced and seen to be free of side-effects, it should be continued for the remainder of the patient's life, which could well be as long as 4 or 5 years even with the presence of such advanced malignancy. Aminoglutethimide inhibits adrenal corticosteroid synthesis and the drug is used mainly for the treatment of metastatic breast cancer after the menopause or oophorectomy. Additional glucocorticoids and mineralocorticoids are required during treatment with aminoglutethimide and adjustments may be required in the dosage of other drugs such as oral anticoagulants and oral hypoglycaemics. The dose is 250 mg twice daily for two weeks increasing to 250 mg four times daily. Bilateral adrenalectomy and hypophysectomy are now rarely performed, although the latter can be carried out relatively non-invasively using an ^{90}Yttrium implant in the tip of a screw which can be inserted into the sella turcica.

Patients with oestrogen-receptor negative tumours respond poorly to hormonal manipulative therapy, but it may still be worthwhile using tamoxifen for a trial period. The other alternative form of treatment for these patients is chemotherapy which has been used in many different combinations. Chemotherapy is, however, most likely to be effective in patients who previously responded to hormonal therapy. Possibly the most useful single agent to date is Doxorubicin (adriamycin) with a response rate of 40 to 50%. These remissions are, however, usually brief. A response rate of over 70% can be achieved with combination chemotherapy using, for example, cyclophosphamide, methotrexate and 5-fluouracil or vincristine.

In premenopausal women with advanced breast cancer androgen administration produces a response in 20% of patients. However, because of the more prolonged and effective remission from oophorectomy this is usually preferred. Oestrogen and androgen therapy are generally of limited value in patients with metastases to the liver, lung or brain. Hypercalcaemia and extensive lung metastases may respond to treatment with corticosteroids.

Pleural effusions are common in advanced breast cancer and are best controlled by closed tube drainage of the chest and intrapleural instillation of a sclerosing agent. Tetracycline (500 mg) in 30 ml of saline is injected into the pleural cavity after drainage of the effusion is complete. The chest drainage tube is then clamped for 6 hours. The procedure may be completed where fluid reaccumulation occurs.

There have been few notable improvements in the management of breast cancer; probably the use of tamoxifen represents the greatest of these in recent years. Undoubtedly those in whom disease is detected at an early stage do better and, to this end, screening programmes have been set up in several cities. The aim has been to detect the carcinoma at a very early, possibly impalpable stage, using clinical examination and mammography. Well women usually over 40 years of age are screened annually using these means. It has yet to be shown, however, that screening either leads to the detection of earlier cancers, or improves the mortality from breast cancer within the screened population. There are no indices which can be used to detect women who run a considerably increased risk of developing breast cancer. As one in 15 women in the United Kingdom develop breast cancer at some stage of their life the identification of a group who had, let us say, a 3- or 4-fold increased incidence of the disease would be desirable. In these patients, who would then have a 1 in 3 or 1 in 4 chance of developing breast cancer, perhaps an argument in favour of prophylactic subcutaneous mastectomy would be raised. No such group has yet been detected.

Case 46

A 36-year-old woman presented with a mole on the left calf. This had been present for several years with recent enlargement, pruritus and bleeding. On examination a nodular lesion 1 cm in diameter was present on the left calf. There were no satellite nodules. Inguinal lymph nodes on the left were appreciably enlarged. Examination of the rest of the body was unremarkable.

Investigations

Electrolytes, liver function tests, haematology, chest X-ray and liver scan all normal.

Questions

What is the differential diagnosis of this skin lesion?
Discuss the surgical management of this patient.

Discussion

The differential diagnosis of a pigmented skin lesion may be summarized as:
(a) benign lesions
    e.g. seborrhoeic keratosis, pyogenic granuloma, sclerosing angioma, keratoacanthoma (molluscum sebaceum), benign naevus (junctional, compound), dermatofibroma and fibroangioma;
(b) malignant lesions
    e.g. malignant melanoma, basal cell carcinoma, squamous cell carcinoma, Kaposi's sarcoma and angiosarcoma.

In this patient the suspicion of malignant melanoma is very high, especially in the presence of enlarged regional lymph glands.

The diagnosis is made by means of an excisional biopsy, removing the entire lesion and, in this patient, the diagnosis of malignant melanoma was confirmed. Three types of malignant melanoma as described by Clark are now recognised. Lentigo maligna melanomas or Hutchinson's melanotic freckles occur in sun-exposed areas on the elderly and have a good prognosis. Superficial spreading

melanomas enlarge by lateral growth and have an intermediate prognosis as lymph node metastases are rare. Nodular
melanomas enlarge by rapid vertical invasion with no intra-
epidermal growth and these tumours have the worst prognosis. Nodular melanomas are usually deep black in colour,
nodular and bleed easily. Lymph node metastases occur
early and blood-stream spread can occur to most organs of
the body.

Two methods of assessing prognosis based on the depth
of tumour growth have been described. Clark described five
stages of vertical growth based on the relationship of the
tumour to the papillary and recticular dermis. Although valuable, this staging system is less frequently used as the
depth of invasion is subjective and considerable variation in
the interpretation exists between different pathologists. Far
more valuable is the staging system described by Breslow.
This method measures the thickness of the tumour in mil-
limetres and is thus a more objective method. Tumours of
less than 0.75 mm thickness (Clark's levels I, II) have a good
prognosis. Tumours of between 0.75 and 1.5 mm thickness
(Clark's level III) have an intermediate prognosis with a
moderate metastatic potential. Tumours greater than 1.5 mm
thickness (Clark's levels IV, V) have a poor prognosis with a
high metastatic potential.

Malignant melanomas are more common on the trunks of
men and the legs of women, as in this case. A region of particularly poor prognosis is the 'BANS' area; upper back, posterior arm, neck, scalp; where metastases occur even with
thin lesions. Women have a 10% survival advantage over
equivalent melanomas in men.

Having made the diagnosis of malignant melanoma by
excisional biopsy, there is considerable controversy over
how the local tumour area should be treated. Treatment of
the regional lymph nodes is a further source of debate.

In this patient, the excisional biopsy revealed a nodular
malignant melanoma of Breslow depth 2.1 mm, that is, a very
poor prognosis lesion. In this situation, wide local excision is
required to prevent local recurrence. The extent of excision
varies between surgeons. With a poor prognosis lesion such
as this a minimum of 5 cm clearance is required and some
surgeons would make the extent of proximal excision 10
centimetres. The excision should extend down to the fascia
and the resultant defect requires skin grafting. Thinner

lesions with a better prognosis require a more localised excision.

The enlarged regional lymph nodes should be removed by block dissection, either at the same time as the wide excision or after several weeks to allow intransit lymphatic metastases to reach the nodes. Considerable controversy exists as to the benefits of prophylactic block dissection of regional nodes. Tumours of intermediate thickness (0.75–1.5 mm) are often associated with microscopic node deposits in clinically negative regional lymph nodes. These patients may well benefit from removal of the draining nodes. Patients with lymph node involvement have an extremely poor prognosis with a median survival of only 24 to 36 months.

Adjuvant therapy in malignant melanoma has been extensively evaluated but its value remains as yet unproven. Immunotherapy may be attempted by means of BCG or *C. parvum* injections. Chemotherapy yields very poor response rates even with the most effective agents available (e.g. DTIC, vindesine, vincristine). Regional perfusion of the isolated limb with melphelan, phenylalanine mustine or radioisotopes may have a role in locally extensive disease. Hyperthermic treatment remains as yet unproven.

Despite these methods of adjuvant therapy, surgery offers the only chance of cure. The expected 5-year survival rate for this patient is a depressing 20%.

Case 47

A 25-year-old man presented with a 6-month history of weight loss, lassitude and generalised pruritus. Recently a swelling had appeared in the left side of the neck.

On examination he was a thin, anaemic, ill-looking young man. Several enlarged lymph glands were palpable in the cervical and supraclavicular regions. There was no evidence of other lymphadenopathy and the liver and spleen were not enlarged. A temperature chart kept over several days showed a moderate intermittent pyrexia.

Investigations

Full blood count demonstrated a normochromic anaemia with a haemaglobin of 10.2 g/dl and an ESR 50 mm/hr. Blood chemistry and liver function tests were normal. Chest X-ray demonstrated widening of the mediastinum. Bone marrow examination was normal.

Questions

What is the differential diagnosis?
Describe the management of this patient.

Discussion

The most likely diagnosis in a young man presenting with lymphadenopathy and gradually increasing lassitude is that of lymphoma. Lymphoma may be either Hodgkin's or non-Hodgkin's in type. Other differential diagnoses to be considered are firstly acute leukaemia, although this should have been recognisable either on the blood film or bone marrow examination. Acute infective causes of lymphadenopathy should then be excluded such as infectious mononucleosis, toxoplasmosis and tuberculosis. Sarcoidosis may occasionally produce similar symptoms.

In this patient, the presence of cervical and mediastinal lymphadenopathy in conjunction with moderate pyrexia and a raised ESR all point to the diagnosis of lymphoma. This should be confirmed by performing a lymph node biopsy of one of the cervical lymph nodes; this should be performed under general anaesthetic as problems may be encountered with exploration of the cervical region under local anaesthesia. In this patient, the diagnosis was nodular sclerosing Hodgkin's disease and the normal architecture of the lymph node was entirely replaced by lymphoma cells.

Hodgkin's disease is a disease of the reticulo-endothelial system characterised by infiltration with lymphocytes, histiocytes and typical Reed-Sternberg cells. Four cellular types of Hodgkin's disease are now recognised according to the Rye classification namely, in order of their increasing malignancy, lymphocyte predominant, nodular sclerosing, mixed cellularity and lymphocyte depleted.

Once the diagnosis of Hodgkin's disease has been made, the next important decision is to stage the extent of spread of the disease. The disorder is staged according to the Ann Arbor classification in stages I to IV, depending upon the number of lymph nodes involved, whether lymph nodes are involved on both sides of the diaphragm and whether extra-lymphatic involvement occurs. In stage I, disease is confined to a single group of lymph nodes. When two separate groups of lymph nodes are involved on the same side of the diaphragm patients are classified into stage II of the disease. Tumours in patients with Hodgkin's nodes on both sides of the diaphragm belong to stage III, and those with widespread disease to stage IV.

In this patient the clinical staging was stage II as both cervical and mediastinal lymph nodes were thought to be involved with Hodgkin's disease. Since treatment is closely related to the stage of disease, the presence of intra-abdominal Hodgkin's disease becomes of critical importance. Abdominal examination rarely demonstrates lymph node enlargement within the abdomen although occasionally inguinal nodes may be felt. Lymphangiograms performed by cannulating a lymphatic vessel in the foot are useful in showing the presence of diseased lymph nodes within the abdominal cavity; however, there is a high percentage of both false positive and false negative results and good radiographs are difficult to obtain in the upper abdomen. Computerized tomography (CT) has recently been utilised to determine the presence of lymphomatous lymphadenopathy within the abdomen and the results obtained show great promise. To date, however, the most important method of determining the presence of intra-abdominal spread of Hodgkin's disease is that of staging laparotomy. Staging laparotomy includes the removal of the spleen, lymph node biopsy of para-aortic, iliac and mesenteric lymph nodes together with liver biopsy. Staging laparotomy alters the clinical stage of Hodgkin's disease in a significant proportion of patients. For example, in patients with known Hodgkin's disease who have an enlarged spleen, in only 80% of these will Hodgkin's deposits be found within the splenic tissue. Of those patients with a normal-sized spleen one third will be found to have Hodgkin's deposits. Patients with stage IV Hodgkin's disease, i.e. Hodgkin's disease involving extralymphatic areas such as the bone marrow, do not require staging laparotomy. In this patient, staging laparotomy revealed no abnormality, thus the final classification was stage II. The presence of fever in patients with Hodgkin's disease is thought to indicate a poor prognosis and symptoms of fever, pruritus and weight loss have been termed B symptoms. The typical undulating fever termed Pel-Ebstein is rarely found.

Treatment of Hodgkin's disease depends almost entirely upon radiotherapy and chemotherapy. Different regimes are employed in different centres. However, mantle radiotherapy is most commonly applied to nodes above the diaphragm. If nodes are present within the abdomen inverted-Y radiotherapy is also carried out. Patients with stage III and stage IV Hodgkin's disease and also all stages of lymphocyte depleted disease require chemotherapeutic regimes also.

The overall prognosis in patients with Hodgkin's disease depends on the pathological classification and the clinical staging of the disease. Patients with stage I lymphocyte predominant or nodular sclerosing Hodgkin's disease have an extremely good prognosis with nearly 100% 5-year survival rates. Those patients with stage IV Hodgkin's disease or those who have lymphocyte-depleted disease have a very poor prognosis. The judicious use of radiotherapy and chemotherapy has, however, radically changed the outlook for patients with Hodgkin's disease and there is now a hope of cure in most patients with this disease. In this particular patient with stage II nodular sclerosing Hodgkin's disease, the chances of cure after radiotherapy are high.

Case 48

A 32-year-old woman presented with a short history of increasing irritability, sweating and weight loss. She had also noticed diarrhoea, menstrual irregularities and increased prominence of the eyes. On examination she was thin and nervous with a heart rate of 120 beats/minute. Both hands demonstrated a fine tremor with marked sweating of the palms. Her eyes showed signs of proptosis with reduced upward eye movement. The thyroid gland was diffusely enlarged with a loud bruit audible over the surface.

Investigations

Normal full blood count and electrolytes. Serum thyroxine was 260 nmol/l and TSH levels were very low. A thyroid scan demonstrated a diffusely enlarged gland with increased isotope uptake. X-rays of the thoracic inlet were normal.

Questions

What is the diagnosis and initial management?
What are the indications for surgery?
What problems are associated with surgery?

Discussion

This patient had thyrotoxicosis and exhibited the classical signs of this condition. The normal initial treatment is medical, by means of drug therapy. The most widely used antithyroid drugs include carbimazole and propylthiouracil which interfere with the incorporation of iodine into tyrosine molecules. These drugs are usually administered for up to one year and are then stopped. Following cessation of medical therapy less than half the patients remain in remission and most require further treatment. If the patient's proptosis is severe an ophthalmic opinion is mandatory as tarsorrhaphy may be required to prevent severe conjunctival and corneal damage. Some patients may require propanolol to reduce marked tremor, sweating and palpitations.

The indications for surgery in patients with thyrotoxicosis may be summarized as: (i) failure to respond to antithyroid medication, (ii) reappearance of symptoms after stopping medication, (iii) severe reactions to medications, (iv) thyrotoxicosis in pregnancy and (v) toxic goitre leading to compression symptoms of trachea and oesophagus.

In some patients the use of the radioactive isotope of iodine ^{131}I has been advocated as treatment for thyrotoxicosis. Usually this treatment is reserved for patients over 45 years of age although there has been a trend towards its use in patients in their 20's and 30's. [131]I is given in a carefully controlled dosage of 80 to 160 µU/g of thyroid and takes 2 to 3 months to achieve full effectiveness. Many patients (3%/year) become hypothyroid and thus require long-term follow-up. The use of the radioisotope of iodine is definitely contraindicated during pregnancy and in children.

The problems associated with surgery in a patient with thyrotoxicosis can be conveniently divided into preoperative; operative and postoperative.

Preoperative preparation is necessary in all patients who require a period of hospitalization. A variety of regimes are described and their basic aim is to reduce thyroid activity and vascularity to a minimum and thus reduce the morbidity of surgery. Propranolol or newer β-blockers with intrinsic sympathomimetic activity are given orally for 1 week preoperatively. These drugs will reduce the heart rate and diminish signs of thyroid overactivity. Many surgeons now use propranolol (20 to 40 mg tds) as the sole preoperative preparation with excellent results. Following surgery the dosage of propanolol is reduced and stopped after 1 week. Antithyroid drugs, such as carbimazole, are often also given to reduce thyroid activity. Aqueous iodine (Lugol's iodine, 0.1–0.3 ml every 3 days) prevents the release of thyroid hormones and is a useful agent in reducing vascularity. It should not be given for longer than 2 weeks since, after this period, a reversed effect on vascularity becomes notable. Tranquillizers such as diazepam can also be effective in calming the patient. Preoperative assessment of the vocal cords must be performed on every patient.

At operation, the use of dilute adrenaline (1:400,000) injected subcutaneously into the neck can be often helpful. Since adequate exposure of the whole thyroid gland is necessary, division of the strap muscles can facilitate the operation. The operation itself consists of removing approximately $\frac{7}{8}$ of the thyroid tissue – leaving approximately 5 g on each side. Care must be taken to preserve both recurrent laryngeal nerves and the parathyroid glands. Meticulous haemostasis and drainage on closure of the wound are vital.

Postoperative problems should be minimal if care is taken with both preoperative preparation and surgery. Respiratory obstruction may occur in the first 12 hours after operation following haermorrhage into the peritracheal tissues, laryngeal oedema or collapse of the trachea with tracheomalacia. Signs of haemorrhage may not be obvious since drains can become blocked; therefore when this complication is suspected the wound should be opened forthwith, the haematoma released and the patient returned to theatre for full haemostasis. Laryngeal oedema and tracheomalacia may require intubation or tracheostomy. Thyroid crisis is now very infrequent and occurs in patients not fully prepared preoperatively. Damage to one recurrent laryngeal nerve results in hoarseness, although this may only be transient. Damage to both nerves is very rare and much more serious as permanent tracheostomy is needed. Surgical trauma to the superior laryngeal nerve will result in loss of strength in the voice and is most noticeable in patients who are singers. Hypocalcaemia often arises following surgery; however, its incidence may be reduced by preserving at least 2 parathyroid glands at operation. This complication is usually only short-term and the patient presents with tingling in the arms and legs with occasional frank tetany. Severe cases are treated with intravenous calcium. Most patients respond quickly to the new vitamin D derivatives (1 α-dihydrotachysterol). Occasionally, patients will require long-term therapy for persistent hypocalcaemia; in this situation, calcium and vitamin D preparations are useful.

Careful clinical follow-up of these patients is needed in all cases. The development of hypothyroidism is frequent and this will require thyroxine supplements. Recurrent thyrotoxicosis is unusual if adequate thyroid tissue is removed at the initial operation. Recurrence is best treated by using the radioisotopes of iodine.

Case 49

A 55-year-old woman presented with a lump in the left side of the neck. She was otherwise asymptomatic. On examination, she was euthyroid with a palpable lump 3 cm in diameter in the left lobe of the thyroid. This lump moved

freely on swallowing and there was no cervical lymphadenopathy. Investigations included normal chemistry, haematology and serum thyroxine levels. X-rays of the thoracic
inlet demonstrated tracheal deviation to the right with a soft
tissue mass in the left neck. Chest X-ray was normal.

Questions

What is the differential diagnosis?
What investigations are helpful in making decisions on treat-
ment?
Discuss the treatment of a solitary thyroid nodule.

Discussion

The presentation of a solitary thyroid nodule in a euthyroid
patient is a common problem facing the general surgeon.
The differential diagnoses are: (i) thyroid cyst (ii) dominant
nodule in a multinodular goitre (iii) benign adenoma and (iv)
malignant thyroid tumour (e.g. papillary, follicular, anaplastic
or medullary carcinomas; or lymphoma).

The initial investigation in this patient should be ultrasonography. With the advent of real time scanners excellent
images of the thyroid gland can be obtained and cystic thyroid nodules can be differentiated from solid tumours. Frequently other areas of nodularity are identified in the thyroid
if a multinodular goitre is present. Solid nodules require further investigation using a thyroid scan. Isotopes of iodine
(^{123}I) or technetium (^{99m}TC) are given parenterally and the
neck is scanned using a gamma camera. The images
obtained may show 'hot' (i.e. increased uptake) areas or
'cold' regions with reduced uptake. Virtually all 'hot' nodules
are benign and may be left *in situ*. All 'cold' nodules must
be removed as 10 to 20% of them will be malignant. Needle
biopsy of a thyroid nodule will often given further valuable
information. Fine needle aspiration cytology is now the technique of choice and the cells obtained may give a clue as to
whether the nodule is benign or malignant. However,
cytology cannot always reliably distinguish between a
benign follicular adenoma and a malignant follicular carcinoma. Moreover, some surgeons are reluctant to rely on
aspiration cytology and advocate removal of all solid

nodules — especially if they are 'cold' on scanning. The use of trucut needles for biopsy is not to be recommended as there is a high incidence of complications and tumour cells may be disseminated along the needle track up to the skin.

A patient with a solitary cystic lesion on ultrasound requires aspiration under local anaesthesia. The fluid obtained should be examined for cytological atypia although most cysts are completely benign. Following aspiration, the patient is reviewed in an out-patients' clinic and, if the cyst does not recur, no further treatment is necessary. Recurrence of a cyst or worrying cytological features are indications for operation. Patients with a multinodular goitre can be left without treatment providing there are no compression symptoms and the thyroid scan is not suggestive of more sinister pathology. This patient had a solid nodule in the left lobe of the thyroid which was 'cold' on scanning. Fine, needle aspiration cytology was indicative of a follicular carcinoma.

The patient with a solitary solid nodule requires surgery and this is mandatory if the nodule is 'cold' on scanning. Little special preoperative preparation other than a routine vocal cord check is needed. At operation, both lobes of the thyroid are inspected as are the lymph nodes around the internal jugular vein. If the nodule is found to involve one pole of a lobe then that pole should be removed with a rim of normal thyroid tissue around the gland. Larger nodules involving one lobe may necessitate almost total lobectomy. Occasionally nodules are present in the isthmus, in which case isthmusthectomy should be performed. Many surgeons now use frozen-section pathological analysis to determine whether the nodule is benign or malignant and to define type of malignancy. If the nodule is benign, no further treatment is necessary. Malignant nodules require further surgery. Other surgeons wait for a full pathological analysis before deciding upon further surgery. In this patient, frozen section analysis demonstrated a follicular carcinoma.

Malignant thyroid tumours can be classified into papillary, mixed papillary/follicular, follicular, anaplastic and medullary carcinomas, and also lymphomas. Each of these tumours has individual features and thus careful pathological analysis is essential.

Papillary carcinoma is the commonest malignancy of the thyroid. It is most frequently seen between the ages of 20 and 40 years and so the patient described here would be unlikely to have this type of tumour. As papillary tumours are often multifocal, a total lobectomy should be performed. These tumours have a tendency for lymph node spread, therefore any enlarged nodes should be carefully removed.

Follicular carcinoma accounts for between 15 and 30% of all thyroid malignancies and tends to occur at a later age than papillary carcinoma. This is the most likely diagnosis in this patient. Many of these tumours are confined to one area of the thyroid although vascular invasion is frequent. Metastases, when they occur, are usually by the blood stream to the lungs and bones. Total thyroidectomy is recommended for follicular carcinoma although a less extensive lobectomy may be sufficient for small non-aggressive tumours.

Many patients have thyroid carcinomas that contain mixed elements of papillary and follicular carcinoma. These patients should be treated by total thyroidectomy.

Anaplastic carcinomas are the most aggressive thyroid tumours and in these patients invasion into the tissues of the neck is frequent. Often the only form of surgery possible is clearance of the trachea; however, total thyroidectomy should be attempted if possible.

Medullary carcinomas are uncommon and there may be a family history of thyroid and other endocrine tumours. They should be treated by total thyroidectomy and removal of affected lymph nodes, although the prognosis is poor.

Lymphomas of the thyroid may occur *de novo* or complicate long-standing Hashimoto's thyroiditis. Total thyroidectomy and postoperative radiotherapy is the treatment of choice.

Following thyroidectomy for papillary, mixed and follicular tumour, a radioiodine scan should be performed to detect residual thyroid tissue or the presence of metastatic disease. If present, these areas must be ablated with ^{131}I. All patients require postoperative thyroxine to prevent myxoedema and also to reduce TSH levels. As some of these thyroid tumours are responsive to TSH, a reduction in the circulating level of this hormone will help to prevent further growth of the tumour.

Recent developments in the treatment of thyroid carcinoma include the measurement of TSH receptors on tumour cells and the use of serial serum thyroglobulin levels to detect recurrence of follicular carcinoma. This patient underwent total thyroidectomy, and a postoperative radioiodine scan failed to demonstrate residual thyroid tissue. She was placed on a maintenance dose of thyroxine and was well 3 years later.

Case 50

A 46-year-old man presented with a typical history of renal colic which was the third episode of renal colic within 1 year. Also, he had recently noticed tiredness, constipation and polyuria. On examination, no abnormality other than renal angle tenderness could be detected.

Investigations

Normal urea and electrolytes Cl$^-$ 112 mmol/l; Ca^{2+} 3.12 mmol/l; PO$_4$ 0.56 mmol/l; alkaline phosphatase 206 U/l. Plain abdominal X-ray revealed stones in the renal pelvis.

Questions

What is the differential diagnosis and how would the diagnosis be investigated?
Discuss the surgical approach to such a patient.

Discussion

This patient has the classical signs of hypercalcaemia. The differential diagnosis of a raised serum calcium can be summarized as: (i) hyperparathyroidism (primary, secondary or tertiary) (ii) metastatic carcinoma involving bone (iii) ectopic parathyroid hormone secretion (iv) sarcoidosis, (v) vitamin D overdosage and (vi) myeloma. Addison's disease, renal failure, milk alkali syndrome, Cushing's disease, acromegaly and pluriglandular syndrome are rare causes of hypercalcaemia.

In this patient the clinical picture is very suggestive of primary hyperparathyroidism (HPT). Hyperactivity of the parathyroid glands is usually related to the presence of a parathyroid adenoma (in 80% of cases) although less common causes are diffuse hyperplasia of the parathyroid glands (in 15% of cases) and parathyroid carcinoma (in 1 to 5% of cases). Most patients with hyperparathyroidism are detected by means of routine serum biochemistry estimations with asymptomatic hypercalcaemia. Renal problems are frequent in HPT and consist of multiple recurrent renal stones and nephrocalcinosis although interestingly these complications rarely occur together in the same patient. Bone involvement is less commonly seen and the classical 'osteitis fibrosa cystica' is now rare. Abdominal pains occur in HPT and these may be due to peptic ulceration, pancreatitis or renal stones. HPT can often be difficult to diagnose with confidence, and a range of diagnostic tests are now available to the clinician. Routine biochemistry will often demonstrate a raised serum chloride in association with a high calcium and low phosphate. Serum alkaline phosphatase is usually elevated, especially when bone involvement is predominant. Since serum parathormone levels are often, although not always, elevated, a more accurate assessment is probably obtained by means of the steroid suppression test. Analysis of the urine will frequently show elevated levels of calcium and nephrogenous cyclic AMP may be detected. Plain X-rays of the hands and skull infrequently demonstrate the classical signs of tufting of the phalanges and the 'pepper-pot' skull. As HPT is often difficult to differentiate from other causes of hypercalcaemia, a series of discriminant scores based on the above tests have been devised.

Patients with disseminated carcinoma and hypercalcaemia most often have a known primary tumour of breast or lung. Plain X-rays will show multiple lesions and the presence of tumour deposits can be confirmed by radioisotope bone scan. These patients will frequently show signs of metastatic disease in other organs such as lung and liver. Myeloma may be excluded by measuring the ESR, protein electrophoresis and by searching for urinary Bence-Jones protein.

The diagnosis of sarcoidosis can be excluded by a normal chest X-ray and a negative Kveim test.

The investigations of hypercalcaemia in this patient were very suggestive of hyperparathyroidism. Several techniques have been suggested as an aid to the preoperative localization of a parathyroid adenoma. Ultrasound scanning is useful in detecting large tumours; however, its accuracy is not yet high enough to suggest widespread use. Small adenomas and a nodular thyroid gland serve to confuse the ultrasonographer. Computerized tomography may be useful in localizing adenomas especially when present in ectopic sites such as the mediastinum. Venous sampling from the neck veins for PTH hormone estimations is rarely used these days as difficulty is encountered in obtaining reproducible results. Recently, technetium and thallium subtraction imaging by radioisotopes has been advocated as an accurate method for preoperative localization.

These patients require little preoperative preparation unless they have severe hypercalcaemia, when intravenous fluids are necessary. All patients should have a preoperative vocal cord check. Intravenous methylene blue may help in the operative identification of parathyroid tissue.

At operation the parathyroid glands are exposed by mobilizing the thyroid gland. The parathyroid glands are usually a pale tan colour and bruise easily on touching. Often they are situated in ectopic sites such as the superior mediastinum, the thymus gland and in the thyroid gland itself. Four glands, two on each side should be identified; however, three or five glands are occasionally present. The most common finding is a single parathyroid adenoma which measures 1 to 3 cm in diameter. In this situation one gland only is affected and the remaining glands are normal or atrophied. When this condition occurs the adenoma should be removed and the diagnosis confirmed using frozen section analysis. In addition, biopsy of half a normal gland should be performed. Where no single adenoma is found the situation of 'four-gland hyperplasia' is usually the diagnosis. All glands are diffusely enlarged and no single adenoma is present. Total removal of three glands and half of the fourth is recommended. The remaining half gland can be left *in situ* in the neck or transplanted into the arm. When a parathyroid adenoma or hyperplasia is not apparent then the operation should be terminated and the diagnosis of hyperparathyroidism re-examined. If the diagnosis is correct the adenoma may well be ectopically located in the mediastinum and thus necessitate thoracotomy.

Postoperatively, these patients may develop tetany especially when bone involvement is severe. Intravenous calcium and calcium/vitamin D tablets are then required. This patient had a single adenoma of the right upper parathyroid gland which was removed at operation. Postoperatively his serum calcium rapidly fell to normal and at 2-year follow-up he had no further renal problems.

Case 51

A 33-year-old man presented with a 1-year history of attacks of headaches associated with palpitations, episodes of sweating and gradually increasing weakness. His blood pressure had been elevated on several occasions and on admission to hospital measured 210/140 mmHg. Examination of the optic fundi confirmed hypertensive changes. The only other abnormal findings on examination were a tachycardia of 110 and pronounced sweating and blanching of the hands.

Investigations

Normal urea and electrolytes, normal creatinine, glycosuria with a blood glucose of 18.6 mmol/l and a normal urea and electrolytes, normal creatinine, glycosuria with a blood glucose of 18.6 mmol/l and a normal full blood count. A chest X-ray demonstrated left ventricular hypertrophy. Electrocardiography showed tachycardia with pronounced hypertensive changes. Intravenous urography was normal. High levels of vanillyl mandelic acid were found in a 24 hour specimen of urine.

Questions

Discuss the surgically correctable causes of hypertension.
Discuss the surgical management of this patient.

Discussion

In most cases of hypertension no demonstrable cause can be found and these cases are termed 'essential hypertension'. The surgically correctible causes for hypertension are (a) phaeochromocytoma, (b) Cushing's syndrome, (c) Conn's syndrome, (d) coarctation of the aorta or (e) renal disease.

In this patient the most likely diagnosis is that of phaoechromocytoma. Such tumours are a rare cause of hypertension, accounting for 0.1–0.2% of all cases. Hypertension is related to the secretion of adrenaline and noradrenaline by the tumour and patients have symptoms related to high blood pressure which can be either paroxysmal or constant. Phaeochromocytomas are usually benign, although 10% are truly malignant. In 80% of patients the tumour is unilateral, in 10% bilateral and in the remainder extra-adrenal e.g. organ of Zuckerkandl, bladder and mediastinum. The diagnosis is only achieved by a high level of clinical suspicion. The group of patients who should be screened particularly for the biochemical abnormalities associated with this tumour include young patients suffering from severe but labile hypertension, and those patients with associated hyperglycaemia or signs of a high metabolic rate.

The most useful test in the diagnosis of phaeochromocytoma is an estimation of the urinary vanillyl mandelic acid (VMA); also known as 4-hydroxy-3 methoxymandelic acid (HMMA). In most patients suffering from phaeochromocytoma the urinary level of VMA is several times greater than the normal level of 8 mg/24hr (40μmol/24hr). When the diagnosis is suspected but the urinary level of VMA is normal several additional tests can be employed. These tests, which must be performed cautiously as dangerous side-effects can result, include blocking tests with phentolamine and provocation tests with histamine. Localization of the tumour is now almost invariably performed by means of computerized tomography. Excellent visualization of the entire retroperitoneal area is obtained. Ultrasonography of the adrenals is also helpful although small tumours may be missed. Intravenous urography may reveal caudal displacement of the kidney. Arteriography may induce hypertensive crises and should be reserved for difficult cases only. Adrenal imaging with $^{131}I - 19 -$ iodocholesterol is not yet in widespread use and its full value remains to be evaluated.

Cushing's syndrome can be excluded by the patient's clinical appearance and by measuring steroid levels in the blood and urine. Renal disease is usually self evident with signs of renal failure. Occasionally renal artery stenosis may require extensive investigation by means of isotope renography, plasma renin levels and selective angiography. Conn's syndrome or primary hyperaldosteronism results in diastolic hypertension with hypokalaemic alkalosis, muscle weakness and fatique, low plasma renin levels and hypernatraemia.

Most phaeochromocytomas require surgical removal. On rare occasions when this is not possible the regular administration of an alpha adrenergic blocking drug such as phenoxybenzamine may be beneficial. Careful preoperative preparation of patients with phaeochromocytoma is essential and requires a period of hospitalization. Alpha-adrenergic blockade is started with phenoxybenzamine in gradually increasing doses until the blood pressure is reduced to normal values. Phenoxybenzamine also reverses the relative hypovolaemia present in these patients, although to achieve this intravenous fluids may also be required. Phenoxybenzamine also helps to prevent blood pressure fluctuations during the operation. Beta blockade with propranolol is reserved for patients with a marked tachycardia and should only be given after alpha-blockade is established.

Operation should be performed through an upper midline incision although the recent advent of accurate computerized tomographic localization may allow a muscle splitting flank incision to be used. Anaesthetic monitoring of the patient by means of a central venous pressure line, an arterial line and cardiography is essential. Changes in blood pressure are usually caused by palpation of the tumour and may be treated by intravenous boluses of sodium nitroprusside or phentolamine. Arrhythmias can be halted by judicious use of lignocaine or propranolol. Profound hypotension can result after removal of the tumour and this is treated by intravenous fluid replacement. The surgeon must examine both adrenal glands as 10% of phaeochromocytomas are bilateral and if no tumour is found the retroperitoneum should be carefully scrutinized. Total adrenalectomy on the affected side is the treatment of choice. Right sided tumours are more difficult to expose, mobilise and excise because of the close anatomical relationship to the liver and inferior vena cava and because of the short adrenal vein which directly enters the inferior vena cava.

Case 52

A 32-year-old female presented with a recent weight gain, facial plethora, bruising and oligomenorrhoea. In addition, she had felt lethargic and complained of generalised muscular aches and pains and weakness. On examination, she was obese with a peculiar distribution of fat such that the limbs were relatively thin compared with the truncal fullness. There was an excessive accumulation of fat around the head and neck area, producing 'moon facies' and a 'buffalo hump'. The patient was plethoric and had purple striae over the anterior abdominal wall and upper thighs. Purpura was present and there were several fresh bruises. There was also an acneiform eruption on the head and neck and partial hirsutism on the upper lip. The blood pressure was elevated at 140/95 mmHg and there was muscular weakness and wasting with some bone tenderness.

The patient had glycosuria, a leucocytosis of $12.5 \times 10^9/1$ and a red cell count of 5.1 million per mm^3. The serum calcium concentration was normal, but the serum potassium was 3.1 mmol/l. X-ray showed generalised bone demineralisation.

Questions

What is the clinical diagnosis?
What laboratory investigations should be performed to confirm this diagnosis?
What is the appropriate treatment?

Discussion

This patient presented with all the clinical features of Cushings' syndrome. The diagnosis of Cushings' syndrome depends on the documentation of increased levels of cortisone in the bloodstream. Cortisol is secreted episodically and there is marked diurnal rhythm. Plasma levels usually peak in the early morning and reach a nadir between 8 p.m. and midnight. It is useful, therefore, to estimate plasma levels at 8 a.m. and midnight. Patients with Cushings' syndrome lose this diurnal variation. Probably the most useful screening test is the determination of urinary free cortisol. Values in excess of 100 μg per 24 hours suggest increased cortisol production. The upper limit of normal for plasma cortisol in the morning is 25 μg and 10 μg in the evening. Plasma ACTH should also be measured. Highest plasma levels occur in the early morning, and lowest in the late evening. Patients with increased plasma cortisol levels, due to adrenal neoplasms, usually have markedly suppressed plasma ACTH levels, whereas those with basophilic pituitary tumours have levels as high as 500 pg/ml. The dexamethasone suppression test is useful in both establishing the diagnosis of Cushings' syndrome and in differentiating pituitary from primary adrenal disease. The patient ingests 1 mg of dexamethasone at midnight and at 8 a.m. the following morning a plasma sample is obtained for cortisol measurement. In normal subjects, or those without Cushings' syndrome, the level should be less than 5 μg/dl. Plasma values above 5 μg/dl suggest hypercortisolism. Following this test sequential low-dose and high-dose dexamethasone suppression tests may be performed with 24-hour urinary specimens collected for 6 days. Failure to suppress cortisol output is strongly suggestive of Cushings' syndrome. A high dose dexamethasone suppression test is useful in differentiating patients with pituitary aetiology of Cushings' syndrome from those with hypercortisolism from other causes. Patients in whom cortisol production is not suppressed following high dose dexamethasone almost certainly have an adrenocorticol neoplasm or an ectopic source of ACTH production. The metyrapone test is useful for evaluating the pituitary adrenal axis and may be used as a complementary test to the dexamethasone suppression test in evaluating the underlying problem in a difficult case. Similarly, the ACTH stimulation test may help distinguish the various causes of Cushings' syndrome biochemically; however, it is less valuable than the former two tests.

A pituitary tumour may be identified by performing radiographs of the pituitary fossa and computerised tomography may be helpful. Adrenal tumours may be identified by ultrasonography, computerised tomography, retroperitoneal pneumography, or arteriography.

The fundamental problem in Cushings' syndrome may lie in the pituitary or in the adrenal gland. Pituitary dependent or true Cushings' syndrome is due to a basophil adenoma of the pituitary. There remains some controversy as to whether or not, in some patients with Cushings' syndrome, there is a hypothalmic aetiology. Adrenal adenomas are the cause of Cushings' syndrome in approximately 20% of patients. These neoplasms are usually solitary and are associated with atrophy of the adjacent non-neoplastic cortical tissue and opposite adrenal gland. Occasionally nodular hyperplasia of both adrenals is present. Multiple adrenal adenomata are very occasionally present. Adrenal carcinoma is a rare but aggressive cause of Cushings' syndrome. It is most common in the third to fifth decade, and the syndrome in these patients usually advances apace. The ectopic ACTH syndrome occurs in approximately 15% of patients with Cushings' syndrome. Here there is no intrinsic abnormality of the pituitary or adrenal gland, rather there is ectopic secretion of ACTH from a distant neoplasm. The lesions most commonly associated with this entity are oat cell carcinoma of the bronchus, pancreatic islet cell carcinoma, and thymic malignancy.

The treatment of Cushings' syndrome is, where possible, surgical. Patients with a basophil adenoma of the pituitary are best treated by transsphenoidal hypophysectomy which is a better approach than the transfrontal approach. Irradiation of the pituitary gland with 5000 roentgens cures about 30% of adult patients and the majority of children with Cushings' disease. Ocular motor palsies, however, occur in up to 10% of treated subjects. Destruction of the pituitary gland can also be achieved by internal implantation of yttrium-90 which is introduced inside a screw using the transsphenoidal approach. Patients with adenoma or carcinoma of the adrenal are treated by adrenalectomy. Medical hypophysectomy has been attempted using bromocryptine, which is a specific activator of the dopaminergic pathways in the central nervous system, apparently enhancing the norepinephrine inhibition of cortisol releasing factor. It is of limited value in the treatment of Cushings' syndrome. Aminoglutethimide inhibits the adreno-cortical secretion of glucocorticoids, mineralocorticoids and androgens. The drug is rather toxic and like bromocryptine does not represent a definitive form of therapy.

Case 53

A 65-year-old man presented to the casualty department with sudden onset of upper abdominal pain radiating through to the back. This was associated with collapse and shock.

Over the preceding few months the patient had com-plained of intermittent pain in the upper abdomen and back associated with occasional episodes of pain in the left leg. He had had a myocardial infarction 3 years previously and had since suffered from significant angina. He was a heavy smoker with a moderate alcohol consumption.

On admission to hospital he was pale and clammy with a blood pressure of 80/50 mmHg and a pulse of 120 beats/minute. Abdominal examination revealed a large tender pul-satile mass above the umbilicus. Both femoral pulses were palpable although distal pulses were absent. A loud aortic murmur was heard over the praecordium and a left carotid bruit was also audible.

Investigations revealed a haemoglobin of 9.6 g/dl with normal blood indices, normal chemistry and markedly ischaemic ECG. The chest X-ray was normal. Abdominal X-ray (AP and lateral views) showed the presence of a large calcified abdominal aortic aneurysm.

Questions

What is your diagnosis?
What treatment does this patient require?
What is the prognosis of this patient both intra- and postope-ratively?

Discussion

This patient has suffered from rupture of an abdominal aortic aneurysm. Often, the diagnosis is difficult, especially if the patient is obese. The presence of collapse and shock are often late events in these patients and an initially symptomatic aortic aneurysm may easily be mistaken for renal colic, pancreatitis or peptic ulcer. The major symptom produced by an aortic aneurysm is back pain. Occasionally embolism arises from the wall of the aneurysm producing peripheral arterial occlusion.

The initial treatment of a patient with a suspected abdominal aortic aneurysm is that of resuscitation. Two large-bore intravenous catheters are inserted into the arm veins. The patient must be cross-matched for at least 6 units of whole blood, oxygen should be administered and a catheter placed into the bladder. Initially intravenous Haemacel or plasma is given followed by blood. After this initial resuscitation, which may well bring the blood pressure to a value of around 100 mmHg, the patient is transferred immediately to theatre for operation. While the patient is still awake, the abdomen and both groins are prepared and the patient towelled for operation. Whilst the patient is being anaesthetised there may be a significant fall in blood pressure. Prophylactic antibiotics are routinely given. When the patient is asleep the abdomen can be opened either through a transverse incision or a long midline incision extending from the xiphisternum to the pubic symphysis. At operation, a large pulsatile mass can be seen in the retroperitoneum and this is associated with significant retroperitoneal haemorrhage. Frank intraperitoneal bleeding is less common and is usually associated with sudden death. The retroperitoneum is opened and the extent of the aneurysm ascertained. A clamp is then placed above the neck of the aneurysm which is usually just below the renal arteries. When serious bleeding occurs which cannot be controlled by the application of a clamp, the aorta can be either compressed at the diaphragmatic hiatus or a Foley catheter can be used to reduce the bleeding. After applying clamps to the aorta and both common iliac arteries the aneurysm is opened and significant lumbar vessels are oversewn. The iliac arteries are carefully inspected and the decision to use either a simple tube graft or a Y graft made. The graft may be inserted from aorta to aorta, from aorta to both iliac arteries or from aorta to both femoral arteries. When the clamps are *in situ* the anaesthetist can proceed with full resuscitative measures and the insertion of central venous pressure and arterial lines. Fresh frozen plasma and cryoprecipitate may be needed to correct clotting problems and control bleeding. Heparinisation is not required in these patients.

Postoperatively the patients must be managed in an intensive care unit and may require ventilation. There are many problems associated with the intra- and postoperative management of these patients. Blood pressure can fall precipitously and may be difficult to control. This should be restored by the use of blood and plasma expanders. The pressure may especially fall low following removal of clamps after the graft is inserted. Circulation to the feet may be difficult to assess when pulses are absent, but cold ischaemic legs may result from either low blood pressure or the presence of emboli in both legs. Embolectomy may therefore be indicated. Renal failure is a significant problem in the postoperative period and is probably related to severe hypotension and interruption of renal artery blood flow. The incidence of renal failure can be reduced by keeping the blood pressure high and establishing a good urine output by the use of drugs such as Mannitol. Dopamine may also be required in the postoperative period both to keep blood pressure high and to improve renal output. Gastrointestinal problems are also encountered; these include duodenal ileus which should be managed by nasogastric intubation and aspiration of gastric and duodenal contents. Ischaemic necrosis of the colon may result from damage to the inferior mesenteric artery which arises from the centre of the aneurysm. Significant ischaemic necrosis leads to the presence of bloody diarrhoea, although mild diarrhoea is often encountered in the postoperative period and this usually settles spontaneously. Spinal cord damage can result from severe hypotension or damage to the major lumbar vessels supplying the lumbar spine. Bleeding problems both during the operation and postoperatively should be controlled by adequate haemostasis and the use of clotting factors, fresh frozen plasma and platelets. The use of fresh whole blood will reduce the seriousness of this problem. Patients with ruptured aortic aneurysms who require more than 10–15 units of blood are at serious risk of developing major problems of postoperative bleeding due to the coagulation deficiency which follows massive blood transfusion.

As this patient was known to have ischaemic heart disease in the past, there was a significant risk of postoperative myocardial infarction. In addition, the presence of a carotid bruit suggested that cerebrovascular accident might also occur. Respiratory problems are especially common in heavy smokers and these can be reduced by the use of antibiotics and physiotherapy. Ventilatory support should be used when necessary.

Late complications in patients having had surgery for aortic aneurysm are those of infection of the graft and broad-spectrum antibiotics must be administered parenterally both during and after the operation. The graft itself may be associated in the long-term with thrombosis, fistula formation or the development of a false aneurysm.

Overall, the mortality of surgery for ruptured aortic aneurysm is around 50%. This compares with the mortality of surgery for an elective aortic aneurysm of less than 5%. The major causes of death in patients with ruptured aneurysms are sudden serious blood loss, severe hypovolaemic shock, myocardial or respiratory arrest and renal failure. Inability to control bleeding during the operation, the presence of an extensive aortic aneurysm precluding the use of grafts and a patient of advanced years (especially over the age of 80 years) are further problems faced by the surgeon. Indeed a significant number of patients die suddenly with ruptured aortic aneurysm before reaching hospital and these are found unexpectedly at postmortem examination.

Case 54

A 56-year-old man presented with a history of increasing claudication in both legs. Pain developed in the thighs and the calves after walking approximately 100 yards. Recently he had also developed pain at rest in the left leg. He was a heavy smoker, smoking 40 cigarettes/day, and had no history of diabetes. For several years he had been mildly hypertensive and was well controlled on beta blockers.

On examination, no abnormality could be found in the neck or in the heart. There was no evidence of an abdominal aortic aneurysm. The left femoral pulse was completely absent and the right femoral pulse reduced in volume with an audible bruit. Pulses distal to this were completely absent. The left leg demonstrated frank ischaemic changes with wasting of the calf muscles, small ulcers on the foot and loss of the pulp of the toes. Sensation and movement were normal in the leg. The right leg showed less marked evidence of ischaemia although two small ulcers were found on the medial side of the right hallux.

Investigations

Urea and electrolytes and creatinine levels were normal. Full blood count and blood glucose levels were normal. ECG demonstrated early ischaemic changes with a sinus rhythm. Chest X-ray and plain abdominal X-ray were normal apart from areas of calcification in both iliac vessels. There was no evidence of aneurysm formation. The brachial pressures measured by means of Doppler were recorded as 140 mmHg. Ankle pressures: left ankle 20 mmHg, right ankle 50 mmHg. Angiography demonstrated gross atheroma of the lower aorta with complete occlusion of the left common iliac artery. The right iliac arteries were extensively involved with atheroma. Circulation in the left leg showed patchy areas of atheroma although a good 'run off' was obtained into the left calf. In the right leg the superficial femoral artery was occluded, but good 'run off' was obtained down the profunda femoris artery.

Questions

Discuss the investigation of patients with suspected peripheral vascular disease.
What surgical manoeuvres would be most likely to improve this patient's circulation?

Discussion

This patient has advanced atheromatous disease of the aorta and both common iliac arteries. This is associated with critical ischaemia in the left leg and advancing ischaemia in the right leg. The situation here demands urgent investigation and surgical therapy. If this is not carried out then irreversible gangrene may result.

Many of these patients have co-existent atheromatous disease in the heart and in the cerebral vessels. It is important to exclude the presence of these lesions by means of ECG and careful examination of the neck arteries. If vascular disease is present within these areas, and is of significance, surgery may also be required to prevent myocardial infarction and cerebrovascular accident. Chest X-ray and lung function tests are essential as the heavy smoking history may also predispose to chronic obstructive airways disease. Analysis of renal function by means of urea and creatinine estimations and creatinine clearance is important as vascular disease can also involve the kidneys and significant hypertension would also cause renal damage.

Many patients with peripheral vascular disease are diabetic and this requires careful treatment if present.

Doppler pressures are a very useful method of determining the degree of arterial insufficiency to the leg. These are entirely non-invasive and are usually expressed as a ratio of leg to arm. Normal leg pressure is greater than that in the arm. A leg:arm ratio of less than 0.5 signifies severe compromise to the vascular supply to the lower limb. In this patient, the Doppler pressure readings indicate very severe reduction in arterial supply to both limbs.

Angiography could have been performed in this patient by transaortic puncture or by transaxillary catheterisation (where the femoral arteries are blocked). Areas of atheroma and ulceration can be identified, as can complete blockage. Later films will demonstrate the adequacy of collateral circulation and the presence of adequate run off in the distal vessels of the calf. Many patients with aorto-iliac disease have co-existing lesions within the femoral arteries particularly at areas such as the adductor hiatus and popliteal trifurcation. This patient had such lesions and these would easily have been missed without the use of angiography. Where run off is very poor in the legs the chances of surgery being successful are extremely limited. In many patients intermittent claudication is self-limiting but the presence of critical ischaemia amounting to rest pain demands urgent surgery.

Having investigated the patient as described and prepared him for operation, two choices of procedure are available. The most commonly utilised method in this country is an aortic bifurcation graft whereby a graft is inserted from the aorta above the area of atheroma to either the iliac arteries or to both femoral arteries. The results of this procedure are excellent if good run off into the distal circulation is present. Poor run off will result in gradual blockage of the graft itself. Long term studies of patients with aortic bifurcation grafts indicate patency rates of above ninety per cent at 5 years in well-selected cases. Blockage of the graft occurs occasionally and this may result from either thrombosis within the graft or neointimal hyperplasia of the endothelial cells lining the graft. Dacron is the material most commonly used for the graft although Goretex is also useful for more distal anastomoses. Endarterectomy is another procedure which is particularly useful for localised disease. However, in this patient with such extensive aorto-iliac disease endarterectomy would probably be unsuccessful because of the extensiveness of the procedure. Where localised disease is present endarterectomy may have excellent success rates. In rare cases patients have one-sided iliac disease and in these a femorofemoral crossover graft may be beneficial. Where significant distal vascular disease is also present further grafts (e.g. femoropopliteal) may be required either at the same time or shortly afterwards.

Postoperative problems in these patients are common and are chiefly related to the patient's associated cardiac, respiratory and renal problems. The problems encountered are myocardial infarction, respiratory failure, renal failure and cerebrovascular accident. In addition, occasional episodes of bleeding may be encountered. Damage to gastrointestinal viscera may also result in significant ileus and colonic ischaemic necrosis. Occasionally spinal cord damage can occur. Whilst performing the operation peripheral embolism must be prevented as this can result in gangrene of the leg, or the presence of showers of multiple emboli may result in 'trash foot'. However, overall the results of aortic reconstructive surgery in patients with good run off are excellent especially if the patient can be persuaded to stop smoking. Certainly continuation of smoking will greatly increase the chances of the graft failing within a short time.

Case 55

A 65-year-old man presented with a 1-year history of increasing pain in the left leg during exercise. Over the preceding few months he had developed marked pain in the calf after walking 100 yards and occasionally experienced episodes of pain at rest. He had also noticed small ulcers developing on the inner aspect of the left great toe. He had been a heavy smoker for many years and 5 years previously had had a myocardial infarction from which he made an excellent recovery.

On examination, his blood pressure was elevated at 160/110 mmHg. His pulse was 80 beats/minute and regular. Examination of the heart demonstrated an aortic sclerotic murmur, and examination of the neck revealed a left sided carotid bruit. Pulses were present in the femoral and popliteal areas of the right leg; however, no foot pulses could be felt. In the left leg the femoral pulse was present with a loud bruit. Distal pulses were absent. The left leg demonstrated signs of chronic ischaemia with loss of hair in the calf and the foot and a shiny appearance to the skin. There was wasting of muscles in the foot and the pulps of the toes were reduced in size. Two small ulcers could be found on the inner aspect of the left hallux and these showed evidence of early infection. Signs of minor ischaemia were present in the right foot also.

Investigations

Normal full blood count, blood chemistry, blood glucose were found. Urine analysis was negative. On ECG an old myocardial infarction with signs of hypertension was demonstrated. The chest X-ray was normal. On the abdominal X-ray no evidence of aortic aneurysm was seen, although calcification could be seen in both aorta and common iliac vessels. Doppler pressures revealed a value of 130 in the arm, 100 at the right ankle and 40 at the left ankle. Angiography showed evidence of marked atheroma in the aorta and both common iliac arteries. In the right leg there was evidence of small blocks in the tibial arteries, although a reasonable circulation was present in the foot. In the left leg the superficial femoral artery was occluded completely in its mid portion, whereas the profunda femoris artery appeared to be patent. Distal run off was good although greatly delayed.

Questions

Discuss the investigations of such a patient with arterial disease.
What surgical manoeuvres are indicated in this patient?

Discussion

In this patient, signs of widespread atheromatous disease are demonstrated throughout his body. He had already experienced myocardial infarction indicating the presence of atheroma in his coronary vessels and the presence of a loud carotid bruit testifies to the presence of disease within the carotid artery. The symptoms of peripheral vascular disease in the legs therefore are one manifestation of widespread atheroma. Intermittent claudication as a symptom indicates a degree of arterial damage. In the long term, however, claudication will often improve with simple measures such as stopping smoking and may require no further treatment.

More urgent signs of vascular disease are those of ulceration, rest pain and frank gangrene. In this patient, the presence of marked claudication associated with rest pain and ulceration indicated a severe degree of ischaemia in the left leg. The results of clinical examination indicated that the patient had arterial disease with vessel narrowing in the femoral artery accounting for the bruit. This is in association with a probable block in the superficial femoral artery. Blocks in this artery usually occur in the adductor canal, and are possibly related to the turbulent blood flow through this area.

The initial investigation of choice is that of Doppler leg/arm pressure ratios since this gives an indication of the degree of blood flow to the limb. In this patient the right leg had a ratio of 100/130 indicating moderate ischaemia which was certainly not limb-threatening at that time. The Doppler ratio in the left leg of 40/130 indicated severe peripheral vascular disease which was certainly limb-threatening. Doppler pressures can be taken at various points in the leg, to indicate the site of blockage. The next investigation of choice is angiography, because this gives a complete map of the arterial circulation to the limbs. Before angiography the patient's blood clotting time must be carefully measured. Angiography can be carried out by Seldinger catheterisation of the brachial artery or the contralateral femoral artery. Occasionally, direct translumbar aortography can be performed. Films are taken of the abdominal aorta and all vessels down to the feet. In this patient widespread atheroma were demonstrated on the films, with particularly marked disease in the left leg. The site of blockage was identified and was found to be in the adductor canal. One important feature to identify on angiograms is that of distal run off. If the vessels distal to an obstruction are poor then there is little hope of successful arterial surgery. In this patient, run off was good and therefore the possibility of successful surgery being carried out was high. In patients with less severe peripheral vascular disease, simple medical measures (e.g. cessation of smoking, the use of leg exercises and the possible use of drugs such as praxilene) may be beneficial. The use of drugs is, however controversial and their benefit is certainly not proven. There is no doubt that stopping smoking will help to prevent progression of disease. The left leg in this patient, however, required urgent surgery to prevent incipient gangrene.

Where small localised areas of tight stenosis are present, balloon angioplasty by means of Gruntzig balloons can be performed. The operation of endarterectomy was originally advocated for superficial femoral occlusions, but this operation has now been shown to have a very high recurrence rate and is therefore no longer performed. The operation of choice is that of femoropopliteal bypass and this is particularly useful where there is good distal circulation. A graft is inserted between the common femoral artery and the popliteal artery. The best graft is that of reversed saphenous vein taken from the ipsilateral leg. Where the saphenous vein is not available or is in poor condition, human umbilical vein (Dardik graft) may be used although patency rates are less. Occasionally, artificial grafts such as Goretex can also be used. Five-year patency rates for patients undergoing femoropopliteal bypass are approximately 70% for saphenous vein and around 50% for artificial grafts.

In situations where the distal circulation is poor and the profunda femoris is narrowed at its origin, the operation of profundaplasty can be performed by widening the origin of the artery with a vein patch. Results following this operation in selected cases are also excellent.

Many surgeons advocate the use of lumbar sympathectomy in patients with peripheral vascular disease, although the use of this operation is debatable where an obvious block can be identified. There is no doubt that sympathectomy will improve the warmth of the leg but its effect on the peripheral vascular disease remains debatable.

Following insertion of a graft into the leg, improved patency rates have been described with the use of long-term Aspirin and Persantin therapy. In many patients, however, little can be done as the peripheral vascular disease is so extensive that a graft cannot be inserted. In these patients, palliative lumbar sympathectomy may be the only operation available. Many of these patients have progressive arterial disease that eventually results in amputation, the level of amputation dependent upon the site and extent of atheroma in the blood vessels supplying the limb.

Case 56

A 64-year-old woman was admitted to hospital with a 4-hour history of pain in the right leg which had been of sudden onset. This pain had developed at rest and had gradually increased in intensity. She had experienced symptoms of parasthesia in the leg associated with difficulty in movement. Over the preceding 6 months the patient had developed signs of ischaemic heart disease associated with mild heart failure. She had been treated by her general practitioner for atrial fibrillation with small doses of digoxin.

On examination her blood pressure was elevated at 160/100 mmHg. There was a fast irregular pulse with a rate of approximately 130 beats/min and no cardiac murmurs were heard. All pulses were present in the upper limbs and the abdominal aorta was normal. Both femoral artery pulses were palpable. The left leg appeared normal with pulses palpable down to the foot. The right leg was cold from the knee downwards with associated pallor and mottling. No pulses could be felt distal to the femoral artery. There was evidence of decreased sensation in the limb with reduced movement.

Investigations

Normal blood chemistry and full blood count were present. Normal chest X-ray. On ECG the presence of fast atrial fibrillation was confirmed.

Questions

What is the diagnosis and the cause of this lady's condition? How should she be treated in both the short and long term?

Discussion

This woman has the classic history and examination findings of an acute arterial embolus. The major sources of such emboli are from the heart in relationship to atrial fibrillation or flutter, valvular heart disease, myocardial infarction and atrial myxoma. Aortic aneurysms and aortic atheroma are common sources of peripheral emboli with a detached thrombus or plaque embolising to the lower limb.

Emboli pass to the lower limb in more than 95% of cases. Less commonly the embolus will pass to the upper limb, the cerebral vessels or to the superior mesenteric artery. When an embolus passes into the lower limb the most common area where lodgement occurs is the femoral artery at the bifurcation into the superficial and profunda femoris arteries. Commonly an embolus may also pass down to the popliteal artery with lodgement at the trifurcation.

Following arterial embolus the patient usually develops sudden pain. The clinical features are pain, pallor, pulselessness, coldness and parasthesiae with paralysis. It is important to emphasise, however, that these changes are often late in developing and may indicate irreversible ischaemia. Indeed, the development of parasthesiae and paralysis almost certainly indicates irreversible ischaemia. The objectives of treatment of such a condition are firstly to control pain, secondly to relieve obstruction and re-establish circulation to the affected area and, thirdly, to prevent further thrombosis with embolisation. The pain in these patients is often severe and careful use of opiates is therefore justified.

Unless the patient is a very poor operative risk, surgery is the appropriate form of treatment. Embolectomy can be performed either under general or local anaesthesia and thus most patients are suitable for such treatment. The classical operation for this particular patient is femoral embolectomy. The femoral artery is exposed in the groin and tapes passed round the common, superficial and profunda femoris arteries. The artery is opened and frequently clot can be removed from this area. Distal clot is removed by passing a Fogarty catheter down the superficial femoral artery. The balloon is then inflated with a small amount of saline and the catheter is pulled proximally. As the lumen of the artery becomes larger, more saline will have to be injected into the balloon. In this way, large quantities of clot are frequently removed from the artery and several passes may be needed to remove all the clot. On the removal of clot back bleeding should occur, indeed the absence of back bleeding is a poor prognostic sign. The profunda femoris artery should then be explored in a similar manner and all clot removed. Heparin solution is usually injected into both profunda and superficial femoral arteries. If there is poor inflow from the common femoral artery the Fogarty catheter is, in addition, passed proximally. Following revascularization of the leg, particularly with long-term ischaemia, severe and profound metabolic acidosis may result; this can cause cardiac arrest. The anaesthetist should therefore be aware of the situation and be prepared to give the patient appropriate quantities of sodium bicarbonate. Some surgeons, following operation, will start the patient immediately on systemic anticoagulant therapy usually by means of heparin followed by warfarin.

The operation of embolectomy is accompanied by a high mortality and morbidity. Mortality is usually related to associated cardiac and respiratory problems and morbidity to long-term ischaemia in the leg. Even following successful embolectomy, some patients will need distal amputation because of irreversible ischaemia. When the patient has had an embolus for longer than several hours, tightness of the muscles in the calf will occur due to oedema. This may result in muscle compartment necrosis and thus worsen the ischaemia. These patients require fasciotomies in the lower limb below the knee to relieve pressure within the three muscle compartments.

In this patient, successful embolectomy was carried out and a large quantity of clot was removed from the superficial femoral artery. No clot could be removed from the profunda femoris.

Following operation, the patient was started on intravenous heparin and oral warfarin. Heparin was discontinued after 2 days. Her dosage of digoxin was then increased and her atrial fibrillation rapidly brought under control. She also required diuretic therapy for mild heart failure.

The long-term results following successful embolectomy are good.

Case 57

A 45-year-old woman presented with a 1-week history of a painful, swollen left leg. This had developed slowly over several days and had been associated with marked swelling of the leg from the groin downwards and bluish discolouration. The day before admission she had also noticed sharp pain in the right chest. She had no relevant past medical history and was not taking any medication.

On examination, she was pyrexial (38.2°C) and had a marked tachycardia. Examination of the chest revealed a loud pleural rub at the right base. The left leg was very swollen with non-pitting oedema and this swelling extended up to the inguinal ligament. The leg was hot with reddish/blue discolouration of the skin. Pulses were impalpable and this was thought to be related to the extensive swelling. The leg was extremely painful to touch and to move. The right leg was normal.

Investigations

Normal full blood and platelet count and blood chemistry. On ECG sinus tachycardia was demonstrated and a chest X-ray was suggestive of a right pulmonary infarction.

Questions

What is your diagnosis?
What methods of treatment are available?
What methods of prophylaxis are available?

Discursion

This woman almost certainly has an extensive deep venous thrombosis in the left leg which was associated with probable pulmonary embolism to the right lung. Thrombosis in a blood vessel is related to a reduction in blood flow, an increase in blood coagulation and endothelial damage (Virchow's triad). Most deep venous thromboses occur in the soleal plexus of the calf and less than 20% originate in the ileofemoral venous segment. There is an increased incidence in women during pregnancy and in patients who are elderly, immobile, obese, suffering from malignancy with thrombocytosis, varicose veins and those who are taking various drugs such as oral contraceptives. Deep venous thrombosis also occurs commonly following operation. Ileofemoral thrombosis is particularly dangerous as there is a very high incidence of fatal pulmonary embolism and extensive thrombosis may lead to venous gangrene of the leg. Following recovery from thrombosis there is a high incidence of postphlebitic syndrome.

Although this patient had the clinical and investigative findings of a classical deep venous thrombosis, thromboses are not always so easy to identify. Investigation of the veins of the leg and the pelvis can be performed by ascending venography. This will determine both the site and size of such thrombi, whether the thrombus extends into the inferior vena cava and common iliac veins and whether such clots are free floating. When the latter occurs, there is a very high chance of fatal pulmonary embolism. It is important to examine the other leg simultaneously since, quite commonly a large coexistent thrombus may be present. Radioactive ^{131}I-labelled fibrinogen can also be used; this technique is particularly valuable in detecting thrombi in the postoperative period and has been used most commonly in clinical studies. Alternatively, Doppler examination of venous blood flow may be used. However, these techniques have poor reliability in the detection of pelvic thrombosis.

The major sequelae of severe deep venous thrombosis are fatal pulmonary embolism, continuing venous obstruction leading to venous gangrene and destruction of the valves of the leg and the blood vessels leading to postphlebitic syndrome.

This patient had a severe deep venous thrombosis and had suffered a pulmonary embolism. Pulmonary emboli are usually detected by means of clinical examination in association with ECG and chest X-ray findings and are confirmed by means of a ventilation/perfusion lung scan, using labelled micromolecules of albumin. Occasionally angiography of the pulmonary vessels will be needed.

Classically, the initial treatment of patients with severe deep venous thrombosis has been by means of heparinisation. The patient is given a loading dose of intravenous heparin and systemic heparin infusion is commenced. The dose of heparin given is carefully controlled by means of blood clotting tests. In the presence of severe deep venous thrombosis heparin should be continued for at least 10 days before commencing warfarin treatment. Oral anticoagulants such as warfarin take approximately 36 hours to become effective and heparin should not be discontinued until oral anticoagulation is fully effective. The dose of warfarin is carefully controlled by means of the prothrombin time and usually takes several days before anticoagulation becomes stable within the therapeutic range. Streptokinase, a fibrinolytic agent, has been advocated for the treatment of severe deep venous thrombosis. This drug has achieved excellent results but should be used with care as severe bleeding can occur in patients on large doses. The antidote for patients with overdosage of streptokinase is epsilonaminocaproic acid. Another anticoagulant that has been used is ancrod which is derived from the Malaysian pit viper. Surgical thrombectomy is occasionally advocated in severe thrombosis; however, there is a high incidence of intraoperative embolism and recurrent thrombosis occurs frequently following surgery. In patients with repeated pulmonary emboli an inferior vena caval filter may need to be inserted. A variety of these is now available and probably the best is that described recently by Greenfield which can be easily inserted under local anaesthetic.

The prophylaxis of deep venous thrombosis and henceforth pulmonary embolism is of critical importance in the postoperative period. A variety of methods have been devised to reduce the incidence of thrombosis as this is a common cause of postoperative mortality and morbidity.

Basically, methods of prophylaxis can be divided into mechanical and chemical types. Mechanical methods that are available are TED stockings, pneumatic leggings, mechanical treadmill, electrical stimulation of calf muscles and perhaps most importantly the use of early mobilization in the postoperative phase. The prevention of pressure on the calves during operation can easily be achieved by elevating the heels.

Chemical treatments available include the use of subcutaneous heparin, intravenous Dextran 70, oral warfarin, aspirin, dipyridamole and various combinations of the above.

In patients at high risk a combination of mechanical and chemical means should be used. Perhaps the most commonly employed system in general surgery today is the use of TED stockings or pneumatic leggings in association with subcutaneous heparin. Occasional cases of major operative and postoperative bleeding have been reported following the use of heparin, although these should not preclude its use in 'at risk' patients.

Case 58

A 65-year-old woman presented with a 2-year history of a swollen left leg. Four years previously she had developed a deep venous thrombosis in the same leg and this was treated with a period of hospitalization and anticoagulation. The anticoagulants had been stopped after 6-months and she had, in the meantime, been well. Over the previous 6 months a large ulcer had developed above the medial malleolus and this had gradually increased in size despite all attempts to treat it by her general practitioner.

On examination, she was slightly obese but otherwise well. The left leg was swollen, particularly below the knee, all pulses were present and there was no evidence of arterial disease. There was no lymphadenopathy in the left groin. Pigmentation was marked below the knee especially on the medial aspect of the leg. The left leg was swollen and no pitting oedema could be demonstrated. A large shallow ulcer 10 cm in diameter was present above the medial malleolus. There was no indication of malignancy. Moderate varicose veins were present in this leg with saphenofemoral incompetence. The right leg was essentially normal.

Questions

What is the diagnosis?
How should this lady be managed?

Discussion

This woman has the classical history and signs of postphlebitic syndrome, although other causes of a swollen leg in association with a leg ulcer must be excluded. The oedema in this patient was not pitting and there was no sign of oedema in the other leg, suggesting that cardiac failure and hypoproteinaemia were not the cause. There was no evidence of lymphadenopathy. It is unlikely that primary lymphoedema could occur in this leg although, obviously, this must be excluded by lymphangiography if suspected.

The pathogenesis of postphlebitic syndrome is related to a damaged calf pump mechanism. Normally the venous pressure in the foot at rest is approximately 80−100 mmHg. On exercise, this pressure drops to around 30 mm and then rises slowly to the resting pressure after 20 to 30 seconds. In the presence of damaged deep valves in the deep venous system, resultant on previous deep venous clinical and subclinical thrombosis the venous pressure remains constant on exercise. There is thus a build up of pressure in the venous system in the lower limb and this is most marked around the perforating veins on the medial side of the calf.

The initial sign of postphlebitic syndrome is the development of an ankle-venous flare above the medial malleolus. This is rapidly followed by skin pigmentation, eczema, liposclerosis and ulceration. The pathogenesis of this condition appears to be related to the escape of fibrinogen from blood vessels because of the high intravenous pressure. Fibrinogen is deposited around the walls of the veins, thus interfering with the transfer of nutrients from the blood to the tissues. The escape of blood and pigment causes the brown pigmentation, and the lack of nutrients in the tissues results in liposclerosis and ulceration.

The treatment of this condition is difficult and it is thus a major cause of morbidity in general practice. In cases where the diagnosis is unclear, ascending phlebography will help to delineate the deep and superficial venous system of the leg. In the postphlebitic syndrome damage to the deep veins will be seen with very few functioning valves left.

The ulcer itself should be managed by antiseptic cleaning as secondary infection will certainly delay healing; desloughing agents are occasionally useful. Compression bandaging and elevation of the limb are essential prerequisites to good healing. In severe cases treatment may require a period of hospitalization with the leg carefully elevated for a period of several weeks. When severe varicose veins are present, they may be surgically treated when the ulcer is healed. The use of antifibrinolytic agents such as stanozolol has recently been advocated in the treatment of postphlebitic syndrome. This medication will help to break down the fibrin cuffs around the capillaries in the leg and thus increase nutrient transfer into those tissues. Good results have been reported in trials using stanozolol in combination with compression bandaging, elevation and careful dressing of leg ulcers. Good treatment, however, demands good patient compliance. In those patients who fail to observe the criteria of leg elevation in association with compression bandaging, little healing of an ulcer will occur.

Case 59

A 37-year-old woman presented with intermittent left renal colic. At first, the attacks were characterized by pain but not by true colic. When the original attack subsided she was left with a dull ache which ultimately resolved. Gradually, the attacks became more severe as a result of which her family doctor organised a plain radiological examination of the urinary tract (KUB) to exclude a urinary calculus. When this X-ray did not show any abnormality he arranged an IVU; this showed 2 entirely normal kidneys, symmetrical in calyceal distribution and opacification. Both renal pelves were normal, and the course and calibre of the ureters showed no abnormality. The bladder outlined and emptied normally.

Subsequently the patient's colicky attacks although infrequent became more severe. She required Pethidine and Buscopan injections to relieve pain. Consequently she was referred for a urological opinion. Apart from a previous appendicectomy, there was no significant past medical history. Physical examination revealed no abnormality, the blood pressure and routine chemical testing of the urine were normal.

Questions

How should the patient be investigated further?
What is the likely diagnosis?

Discussion

The history and the clinical evidence were suggestive of a renal abnormality. During an attack of pain the patient also complained of tenderness in the left renal area, although previously she had never been examined at the time of an attack. She had had no back injury nor was there any suggestion that she had a spinal abnormality. The plain X-ray of the urinary tract (which also doubled as a spinal X-ray AP view) was normal. There was nothing to suspect a bowel disorder and a barium investigation would have been inappropriate.

Since the patient might have been suffering from intermittent hydronephrosis a high dose urogram (which was essentially normal) and a standard renogram (which showed the function in both kidneys to be equal and normal) were carried out as control procedures. The patient was then invited to contact us when she developed the next attack of renal colic since it was our intention to arrange an urgent intravenous urogram IVU. In due course the patient presented in severe pain and a standard urogram was carried out. The initial films were unremarkable, but after 15 minutes the left renal pelvis began to distend. At 90 minutes, the renal pelvis had enlarged to the size of a tennis ball and the calyces were slightly dilated. The left ureter did not show. This IVU had increased the patients symptoms, thus it was necessary to prescribe Pethidine during the test for relief of pain. During the next attack, a standard renogram was arranged which showed an entirely normal right kidney. However, the pattern of the excretion of the left kidney function was obstructive showing no evidence whatsoever of excretion of the isotope. These two investigations performed during attacks of colic confirmed the diagnosis of intermittent left hydronephrosis.

Neither an ascending ureterogram nor a retrograde pyelogram were contemplated on this woman in view of the normality of the original IVU. These would not have provided us with any further information; however, it was extremely advantageous to be able to carry out the two confirmatory investigations during painful attacks on an outpatient basis. This was not easy to make provision for, but sufficient concern about the discrepancy between her symptoms (which seemed to be genuine) and the normality of the basic investigations warranted such measures.

Once the diagnosis had been made, it was recommended that the patient undergo an exploratory operation of the left kidney with a view to carrying out a left pyeloplasty. Since the patient was suffering from intermittent hydronephrosis, it was particularly unlikely that we would be operating during an attack of pain; therefore, on the morning of operation an intravenous infusion was set up to keep the patient well hydrated. Indeed, the drip rate was increased at approximately the same time the premedication was given in the hope that the abnormality would be seen at surgery.

The operation was performed through a left loin incision with subperiosteal resection of the twelfth rib. There was no abnormality of the perirenal tissues and the kidney substance looked entirely normal. The renal pelvis was a little full because the patient was receiving an IV infusion but there was no gross hydronephrosis. The ureter looked normal and there were no lower polar vessels. The anaesthetist was requested to increase the infusion rate and the patient was given a diuretic after which the renal pelvis distended significantly. An Anderson–Hynes pyeloplasty operation was then started. The ureter was divided below the pelvi-ureteric junction after which no urine emerged from the distended renal pelvis. The renal pelvis was then opened and urine allowed to drain away freely, during which time a piece of tissue the size of a match head floated out with the urine. This looked like a 'blob' of mucus but was sent for histological examination. The standard Anderson–Hynes pyeloplasty was completed and the removed pelvi-ureteric junction sent for microscopic examination. On this occasion, the anastomosis was not protected by a nephrostomy tube, but a tube drain was placed down to the kidney bed and the wound closed with absorbable sutures.

While the patient was making an uneventful postoperative recovery, the pathology department confirmed that the piece of tissue that seemed to be free floating in the renal pelvis was actually a transitional cell carcinoma. Although the resected segment had been sent for electron microscopic examination, some of this tissue was also subjected to standard histological investigation and a focus of transitional cell carcinoma was identified at the pelvi-ureteric junction. In due course the electron microscopic examination of the renal pelvis revealed unremarkable collagen distribution.

Questions

What should the future management of this patient be?

Discussion

The intermittent hydronephrosis resulted from the small piece of tissue at the pelvi-ureteric junction. This was occasionally 'ball valving' into the upper ureter and causing an obstruction, giving rise to colicky pain and hydronephrosis as shown on the IVU and renogram investigations performed during colic attacks. The Anderson–Hynes pyeloplasty which was carried out because of intermittent hydronephrosis was arguably curative but, since transitional cell carcinoma is a reflection of an unstable urothelium a silent recurrence may develop in the renal pelvis which might be difficult to diagnose afterwards; thus the distortion following surgery might make reading IVUs unreliable. Neither would it be appropriate to pass a ureterorenoscope up through the bladder and ureter and across the pelvi-ureteric junction that had undergone surgical revision in an area where carcinoma existed. The possibility of missing a small lesion (perhaps the size of a match head) would be high.

The patient was therefore advised by us to undergo an orthodox left nephro-ureterectomy. She was unable to cope with the idea that she might have a cancerous disease and was very willing to take our advice. Several weeks later, a left nephro-ureterectomy was performed through the original left loin incision and an oblique lower abdominal incision. When the kidney had been disconnected from the renal pedicle, it was placed in a large surgical glove which was tied around the ureter and pushed retroperitoneally down into the anatomical pelvis. The upper wound was then closed, the patient turned flat and through the lower incision the distal end of the ureter was disconnected with a cuff of bladder epithelium. Thus, the specimen was removed *en bloc*. Prior to this, a cystoscopy had been carried out to exclude transitional cell disease in the bladder.

The patient currently remains well and symptom-free several years post surgery, undergoes annual review cystoscopies and is subjected to an intravenous urogram every 3 years. The histology of the removed nephro-ureterectomy specimen was entirely normal and this kidney was subjected to serial sectioning and histological review. The programme for the future is to continue to carry out review cystoscopies and perform IVU's at 3-yearly intervals.

This presentation of transitinal cell carcinoma at the renal pelvis is quite unusual. Renal pelvic carcinomas usually become obstructive, the condition becomes progressive and unremitting and frequently presents with haematuria. At no stage did this patient have any suggestion of haematuria on microscopy. It is distinctly possible that if we had not subjected her to investigation during attacks of pain she may well have been labelled a 'functional'. The attacks of pain were quite severe and clearly occlusive and she was requiring a substantial amount of pethidine and Buscopan to relieve them; this eventually may have become addictive. Other similar cases of intermittent hydronephrosis have been seen by us but she is the only one in which a diagnosis of transitional cell carcinoma has been made with an initial normal standard urogram.

Most presentations of intermittent hydronephrosis occur in teenagers or young adults, with a classical onset of pain in the affected kidney on waking in the morning. This onset of pain occurs frequently in patients who have been drinking several pints of fluid, such as beer, the night before. The kidney becomes obstructed because of the enforced diuresis during the night and when the patient wakes in the morning the pain is present. As the day progresses the symptoms usually abate. In such people a standard IVU may be normal, and the intermittent nature of the obstruction may only be demonstrated either by an IVU at the time of the attack of pain or a stress renogram (which is carried out by giving the patient some fluids and frusemide before the isotope). However, not all intermittent cases merit surgery. If the patients are able to abstain from a high fluid intake over a short period of time, the likelihood is that surgery will be avoided and that their renal function will be preserved at the presenting level. Some cases of intermittent hydronephrosis occur in fit young adults who play aggressive sports such as squash, become dehydrated and then rehydrate themselves afterwards. If the fluid intake continues for some hours then symptoms may arise before retiring to bed; thus the patient may think the symptoms are related to exercise. This also happens in those who present with pain in the kidney in the morning on waking and because of this, the initial diagnosis tends to be one of a musculoskeletal disorder. However, when questioned about fluid intake prior to an attack, the clue to the patient's diagnosis is revealed.

Case 60

A 58-year-old female suffering from diabetes and severe rheumatoid arthritis, with a previous history of urinary tract calculous disease, presented with severe left renal pain. This woman suffered from maturity onset diabetes which was controlled by diet and an oral hypoglycaemic agent. She had suffered from rheumatoid arthritis for many years during which she had taken steroids to stem the progression; this disease mainly affected her wrists and hips. She was also taking a considerable amount of oral analgesics. Several years previously, the patient developed diabetes and, before the rheumatoid arthritis had become dominant, she had undergone an open removal of a left renal calculus. She had long since ceased to be followed up at the Urology Clinic as she was attending the Rheumatology Clinic regularly. A plain X-ray of the abdomen taken several years previously revealed the presence of a small recurrent calculus in the lower pole of the left kidney but, as this was asymptomatic, it had been decided to leave it alone.

Examination revealed a woman of small stature who was clearly handicapped by her rheumatoid arthritis which limited use of all four limbs. She was also obese and stooped. The left renal area was tender but bimanual palpation of the abdomen did not reveal a palpable mass.

The preliminary investigations revealed the presence of a calculus opposite the transverse process of 3rd lumbar vertebra; additionally, an IVU confirmed a normal right urinary tract, but a totally obstructed left kidney with a nephrogram appearing after 1 hour. Her urea and electrolytes were normal but her creatinine was slightly raised. Her haemoglobin was 11.2 g/dl, WBC normal and ESR was 50 mmh. Her blood pressure was 160/100 mmHg and she was in sinus rhythm and had a slight tachycardia. She had a low grade temperature on admission.

The patient was requiring large doses of pethidine to relieve the severe pain that she was experiencing from her obstructed kidney. She was already on oral analgesics for her arthritic pain.

Question

What are the treatment options open to the urologist?

Discussion

Ideally, the urologist would like to be able to offer his

patients the choice of either Extracorporeal Shock Wave Lithotripsy (ESWL), percutaneous nephrostolithotomy (PEN), or open surgery in appropriate cases. Presently, however, few urologists in the UK can offer their patients all three treatment options. This woman's calculus, which was 1.5 cm in diameter and mainly round and smooth, had no real possibility of passing spontaneously; thus some form of urological intervention was required.

Open removal of the recurrent left ureteric calculus would be the least attractive option for this patient. Since she was a mild diabetic, suffered from severe rheumatoid arthritis which required large doses of steroids and because she had already undergone open surgery on her left kidney, she did not present as an ideal candidate for further surgical removal of the calculus. Those patients who are on large doses of steroids and who develop obstructed kidneys from calculous disease are at risk of developing an infection in the obstructed kidney which, combined with the high steroid doses, may prevent the upper urinary tract from healing and after surgery cause persistent urinary fistulae to occur. We had no evidence that this woman had an infected kidney at the time because her urine was sterile (there was no urine being produced by the obstructed kidney), her temperature was just above normal and her white count was not raised.

Extracorporeal Shock Wave Lithotripsy (ESWL) is not universally available and, had it been available in our hospital, she would have been an ideal candidate for treatment. She could without any difficulty have been given an anaesthetic and lowered into the water bath for treatment on a Dornier machine. The stone could easily have been visualised and once it had been pushed back into the upper ureter (performed at a preliminary cystoscopy and retrograde manipulation of the stone) the calculus could have been easily disintegrated with the patient passing the fragments with little difficulty. All that would be required would be to increase her steroids during the procedure and to treat her with an antibiotic. In addition, her diabetes would be very unlikely to be upset by an ESWL procedure.

The third option available is a percutaneous nephrostolithotomy (PCN). This is preferable to open surgery but not as satisfactory as ESWL. The patient is given a scar approximately 1.5 cm in length and undergoes minimal surgical manipulation. Because of the reduced amount of tissue disturbed at surgery a fistula should not persist afterwards even in someone on steroids. The percutaneous needle is placed through the renal capsule and renal substance into a calyx to allow access to the stone in the renal pelvis. Thus an open surgical procedure is avoided, obviating the possibility that the renal pelvis might not heal afterwards. The percutaneous renal track is more likely to heal satisfactorily by the closure of the renal substance over the track as soon as the nephrostomy tube has been removed.

The patient was investigated as soon as she arrived in the hospital and by the end of the same day her general state had been assessed and a firm diagnosis had been made. Because she was a mild diabetic, it was decided that the next morning she would be offered a PCN since the nearest ESWL facility was over 200 miles away and an emergency ESWL procedure could not be organised at short notice.

With her premedication she was given an extra dose of steroids and also an intravenous bolus of gentamycin and flucloxacillin. A preliminary cystoscopy was performed in order to introduce a ureteric catheter up the left side to flush the calculus back into the renal pelvis. The preliminary cystoscopy was achieved with the patient lying flat. Her hip condition would not have easily allowed the lithotomy position, but since the patient was female it was quite easy to catheterise the ureter with her lying flat. A guide wire was passed up the left ureteric orifice into the upper ureter; over this an angiographic catheter was passed. Saline was then flushed through the catheter into the upper ureter onto the impacted stone which was dislodged and displaced into the renal pelvis. A two-way pelvic-ureteric junction occlusive balloon catheter was then introduced into the ureteric orifice and the balloon inflated below the level of the pelvi-ureteric junction to prevent the stone from returning to the ureter. Through the other catheter channel some urografin and methylene blue were injected into the renal pelvis and calyceal system. This had the effect of opacifying the collecting system and allowing the radiologist to confirm when he has entered a calyx with his renal puncturing needle. A catheter was then put in the bladder to secure the ureteric catheter in place. The patient was then turned over onto her face and positioned so that the left side of her body was raised 15° off the table.

Under image intensification, the radiologist selected a

calyx for puncture and dilated the track with fascial dilators up to size 30F; next an Amplatz sheath was placed over the widest dilator. The urologist then introduced a nephroscope down the Amplatz sheath positioned across a calyx and reaching into the renal pelvis. The stone was then easily seen; it was too big to grasp, therefore it was disintegrated by using an ultrasound probe which was passed down the operating element of the nephroscope. The ultrasound probe had the facility of sucking out the fragments as they were disintegrated. Some of the larger fragments were then extracted with special forceps, and throughout the procedure the renal pelvis was irrigated with normal saline. When the urologist was satisfied that all the fragments had been removed, the nephroscope was withdrawn and a nephrostomy tube placed down the Amplatz sheath. A nephrostogram was carried out to ensure that it was positioned correctly and that there was no extravasation. The Amplatz sheath was then removed, the nephrostomy tube fixed in place by a skin stitch and attached to a urine collecting bag.

After this procedure the bladder catheter was left in for 24 hours. The patient was kept on an appropriate dose of steroids and antibiotics and the next day the nephrostomy tube was clamped. It was removed 24 h later, resulting in minimal leakage from the nephrostomy site. Patients are usually discharged the next day. In this particular case, the patient was kept in hospital for a few days while her steroids were reduced and in order to complete the course of gentamycin. Her diabetes was unaffected by the procedure, her rheumatoid condition was not adversely affected by the PCN and the stone was removed through a small incision.

The total hospital stay was less than 1 week. Instead of having her old scar reopened with the attendant problems in someone who is a diabetic taking steroids, she was rendered stone free and pain free by a small incision in the loin.

Case 61

A 50-year-old man suffering from Albers-Schonberg disease (osteosclerosis fragilis) presented with low back and sciatic pain together with tiredness. Two months previously he had suffered from an attack of herpes zoster on the abdominal wall. More recently he had complained of a vague ache in the right loin and frequency of micturition. The frequency was most noticeable during the attack of herpes zoster. He denied haematuria. He had no other lower urinary tract symptoms and there was no true polydypsia. His appetite was good and he had not lost any weight but there was some looseness of the bowels. He thought that his stools were slightly paler than usual but they did not float. He had undergone an operation for a prolapsed disc 13 years previously and subsequently injured his back playing squash which had never recovered completely. On questioning, he admitted to headaches of recent onset; no further information of value was yielded.

Examination revealed a man of large stature who had a slightly sallow complexion possibly consistent with uraemia. Vague epigastric resistance but no other physical abnormality was present. His blood pressure was 160/90 mmHg sitting upright. There was no lymphadenopathy, but rectal examination revealed a small benign prostate and routine chemical testing of his urine was normal.

The initial investigations showed that, in addition to his urine being chemically normal, it was also bacteriologically normal. His haemoglobin was 12 g/dl, white cell count 8900, ESR 9 mm and urea 17.6 mmol/l and creatinine 370 mmol/l. Total protein was 67 mmol/l, serum calcium 2.52 mmol/l and γGT 40 mmol/l.

Our initial assessment was that his low back pain and sciatica might have been related to his previous surgery and injury to his back. The frequency of micturition may have been accounted for by the herpes zoster which might well have affected his bladder in the acute phase, as the distribution of the shingles was along the line of T12. The Albers-Schonberg disease was thought to be unrelated to his biochemical findings and there was nothing to suggest that he was suffering from polycystic kidney disease.

Questions

How does one proceed to investigate this problem?

Discussion

His chest X-ray showed neither evidence of active lung disease nor metastases, but increased bone density consistent with Albers—Schonberg disease was present. The plain X-ray of the urinary tract (KUB) was non-contributory and there did not appear to be any abnormal distribution of bowel shadows. Although the patient was uraemic we arranged an IVU which showed that there was very poor function in the left kidney, and the right kidney was essentially non-functioning but appeared on the nephrogram to have a mass arising out of it. Although some contrast was seen in the bladder on the later films, no real information was obtained about the course and calibre of the ureters.

We now had a patient who had presented in renal failure and whose preliminary investigations gave no reason for the failure except that there was possibly a mass arising out of the right kidney but that in itself would not explain the poor functioning of the left kidney.

Questions

What is the next line of investigation?

Discussion

On reviewing the case we were a little suprised to find that the urine test was chemically normal, that there was no suggestion of pus cells or red cells in his urine, that the sedimentation rate was normal and yet he was uraemic. Some form of retroperitoneal pathology such as retroperitoneal fibrosis might account for the findings but would not explain the apparent mass arising from the right kidney. We proceeded to non-invasive tests, namely an ultrasound examination of the upper abdomen and renography. The ultrasound investigation suggested that there was a mass either arising from the right kidney or, alternatively, arising on the posterior abdominal wall and involving the right kidney and also surrounding the inferior vena cava. This, however, did not explain the poor function in the left kidney. A renogram was carried out which showed that the left kidney had a prolonged isotope transit time with a significantly reduced excretory phase. The right kidney was hardly functioning at all.

By now our attention was moving away from a primary renal condition and we felt that some form of retroperitoneal pathology might account for the investigative results. A cystoscopy was then carried out which showed an entirely normal bladder and bilateral ascending ureterograms were performed. The course and calibre of both ureters were entirely normal and on the right side the collecting system was well shown and all the calyces were filled. On the left side, an entirely normal pelvicalyceal system was present. An examination under anaesthesia of the abdomen revealed an epigastric mass but neither kidney nor the liver was identifiable.

The presence of conventional retroperitoneal fibrosis such as might encroach on the ureters and explain his renal failure had now been excluded. Several investigations were repeated and found to be essentially unchanged, in particular the differential white cell count was normal. The neutrophils were 72%, lymphocytes 26% and monocytes 2%. All of these initial investigations were carried out over the course of 1 week.

This patient's renal failure and the mass in the epigastrium were still inexplicable. His right loin discomfort was probably related to the right renal mass and the backache could have resulted from some retroperitoneal disease such as a lymphosarcoma. At this stage we felt it was entirely justifiable to proceed to an arteriogram and a CT scan. A right renal selective arteriogram showed no evidence of tumour circulation on the right side such as one might find in an adenocarcinoma of the kidney. The distribution of the blood vessels, however, was rather curious and there seemed to be an abundance of them. On the left side, the arteriogram was entirely normal. An injection of contrast medium into the aorta showed that the coeliac axis and mesenteric systems were entirely within the normal range. This investigation, therefore, was in no way diagnostic. Apart from possibly excluding an adenocarcinoma of the right kidney (which again would not have explained the poor function of the left kidney), it did not help with the diagnosis.

The CT scan revealed osteosclerosis in the lumbar vertebra but also two lytic areas in the vertebral body of L2; however, it was not thought that this was due to metastatic disease. An intravenous injection of contrast medium was given at the same time as an inferior vena cavagram was carried out under CT imaging. The calyceal pattern on the right side was not shown but there was considerable delay in excretion from the left kidney where mild hydronephrosis was present. The inferior vena cava seemed to have a soft tissue mass within it; this was concluded to be a large right-sided tumour associated with extensive para-aortic and para-caval lymphadenopathy with a malignant extension in the inferior vena cava. However, the delay in excretion of contrast within the left kidney was still unexplained.

All the data was now reviewed and there was obviously conflicting evidence. It was clear that there was glandular enlargement in the upper abdomen particularly in the epigastric area and this would have explained the epigastric resistance and there seemed to be evidence of enlarged lymph nodes around the aorta and inferior vena cava, yet there was no lower limb oedema. On the CT scan the right kidney was considered to have a hypernephroma adreno-carcinoma and yet the retrograde examination of the collecting system suggested that this was entirely normal, which would not be consistent with the diagnosis of adreno-carcinoma.

The only non-invasive technique left to us was an nuclear magnetic resonance (NMR) investigation. This showed an extensive retroperitoneal mass extending over approximately 21 cms to below the aortic bifurcation and passing through the diaphragm into the retrocrural and para-aortic region. The mass filled most of the left side of the abdomen and crossed over the right side, with extensive anterior displacement of the inferior vena cava, and, to a lesser extent, the abdominal aorta. There did not appear to be any spinal involvement. Clear definition of renal structure, however, was not apparent probably because of displacement by the mass.

At this stage, we were considering that retroperitoneal pathology of the lymphosarcomatous type was present in the upper abdomen, which was affecting the circulation to both kidneys. Although the NMR investigation suggested that most of the tissue was on the left side, there was still some doubt as to whether there was an intrinsic lesion in the right kidney or not; thus it was decided that the right kidney ought to be explored. A laparotomy in conjunction with exploration of the right kidney would be appropriate and so the patient was positioned at a 45° angle to the table. A curvilinear incision was made over the lower end of the 12th rib across the abdomen. The peritoneum was opened but there was no free fluid in the peritoneal cavity. The left kidney was tense and the tip of the spleen was felt. On the right side, the kidney itself was involved in a mass which reached as far up as the under surface of the diaphragm but the liver was clear of the mass. The mass itself seemed to be fixed to the psoas muscle posteriorly and stretched across the midline, this being consistent with the NMR findings. The basic impression was that this man was suffering from a retroperitoneal disease which was impeding the circulation to both kidneys and also involving the right kidney. The right kidney did not appear to be intrinsically carcinomatous. The appearance, however, was grossly abnormal and it was decided to perform a biopsy in the lower pole.

This was performed and a wedge of tissue about 2.0 × 2.0 cm and 0.5 cm thick was removed. The kidney was very vascular, as were all the surrounding tissues. The tissue was sent for frozen section and, before the abdomen was closed, a provisional diagnosis of a lymphomatous condition involving the kidney was suggested. The subsequent paraffin sections confirmed the presence of a diffuse cellular infiltrate consistent with a malignant lymphoma. Although the overall features were of a non-Hodgkin lymphoma, the presence of eosinophils in the infiltrate was suggestive of a possibility of Hodgkin's disease.

Now that the tissue diagnosis had been made, no further surgery was appropriate; thus he was referred for a oncological opinion. Initially it was decided to treat him with chemotherapy and to withhold radiotherapy until the response to the chemotherapy had been assessed. He had an initial induction course of vincristin, adriamycin and prednisolone. He withstood this well and shortly afterwards was given a consolidation course of cyclophosphamide. A CT scan at this stage showed considerable improvement in the previously-noted adenopathy. Although not all the disease had been destroyed there was a return of function in the right kidney and by now his creatinine and urea levels were falling.

Four months after the laparotomy another thoraco-abdominal CT scan was performed; this showed substantial mass disease in the upper right retroperioneum with only a little lymphadenopathy on the left side of the aorta. The right kidney and psoas muscle were clearly involved in continuity and on the right side there was still considerable disease. In an inferior direction the disease persisted as far as the vascular bifurcation but there was no evidence of iliac lymphadenopathy. The mesentry appeared clean. Clinically there was no discrete mass in the abdomen but there was fullness on the right side. He was therefore given a radical course of radiotherapy and at the end of this the fullness in the right side of the abdomen had largely subsided.

Over the next 12 months he remained reasonably well and was able to return to his employment. His haematological and biochemical estimations were essentially normal and, although he felt tired, he had no specific symptoms. However, 18 months after the initial diagnosis was made he complained of an irritating cough and vague abdominal pains.

Clinically, the only abnormality was a right pleural effusion which was confirmed by a chest X-ray which also showed there was a paraspinal mass at the thoracic level. Aspiration of the pleural fluid revealed abnormal lymphocytes consistent with the recurrence of non-Hodgkin lymphoma. In view of this, he was restarted on chemotherapy with vincristin, adriamycin and prednisolone in an initial induction course over a 6-week period.

Following this he was quite well and there was evidence that the treatment had reinduced a remission. His Prednisolone was reduced and then he was started on a consolidation course with cyclophosphamide and Etoposide. The pleural effusion disappeared completely and the chest X-ray was clear. He had 2 further courses of consolidation therapy. He was now on a maintenance treatment of cyclophosphamide and methotrexate weekly and mercaptopurine daily; the dose of treatment being adjusted according to his blood count.

At present, over 2 years after the initial presentation and diagnosis he remains well and is clinically free of disease, his chest X-ray is normal, both kidneys are functioning, but he remains on maintenance chemotherapy.

This man presented with vague symptoms and it was only by carrying out the biochemical analysis that there was any indication of what the diagnosis might be. He was diagnosed as having chronic renal failure but the cause turned out to be extrarenal. He had no true lower urinary tract symptoms apart from his frequency which was probably accounted for by the herpes zoster affecting the T12 segment. This may have given rise to changes inside the bladder mucosa, sometimes seen in these situations.

This patient was investigated in a step—wise fashion, starting with the conventional urological investigations, including a chest X-ray and a KUB, followed by an IVU. This was performed, despite the fact that he was in renal failure, and was entirely justified. When a mass was discovered, and also poor function, it was reasonable to proceed to ultrasound examination of the abdomen, which actually underestimated the amount of disease in his upper abdomen and tended to suggest that he had a tumour of the kidney. Renography was performed merely to ascertain the differential function on both sides since the IVU is unreliable in providing information about function. The interpretation of the renogram was that there was no obstruction to the outflow on either side, but that there was poor uptake of the isotope in both kidneys, the right kidney hardly functioning at all.

It was important to exclude retroperitoneal fibrosis and the simplest way of doing this was to carry out a cystoscopy and ascending ureterograpy. This showed 2 entirely normal ureters which negated the presence of any disease on the back wall affecting his ureters. Subsequently an arteriogram was justified on the basis that more knowledge about the renal arteries on both sides was needed; also, by carrying out a bolus arteriogram, information about the rest of the vasculature in the abdomen could be obtained. The vasculature was essentially normal although some of the vessels were somewhat displaced. This procedure did not provide us with a diagnosis. The CT scan tended to suggest there was an adrenocarcinoma in the right kidney together with lymph node enlargement around the kidney, the aorta and inferior vena cava. Only by nuclear magnetic resonance scanning was the full extent of the pathology in his abdomen defined; however, this again did not provide us with a diagnosis. It required an exploratory laparotomy to get a tissue diagnosis after which treatment was planned.

It could be argued that many of the investigations might have been avoided if the patient was subjected to an operation in the first instance after it was found that he had a mass in the right side and poorly functioning right kidney. It would certainly have provided us with a tissue diagnosis earlier than it was obtained but would not have led to a plan of treatment afterwards. The patient would still have needed a CT scan, and this is the way he has been monitored ever since. The use of an NMR scanner was a luxury but was very useful to define the exact limits of the disease in a way that the CT scanner did not.

This man's prognosis is uncertain but it is encouraging that 2 years after diagnosis he remains well and virtually symptom-free, although he is on maintenance chemo-therapy.

Case 62

A 63-year-old man presented with intermittent haematuria. Physical examination revealed no abnormality apart from a somewhat enlarged benign prostate. His urine contained red cells but was sterile, a chest X-ray and IVU were entirely normal apart from a small amount of residual urine in the bladder at the end of micturition. At cystoscopy the bladder mucosa was completely normal but there was a large vessel coursing over the bladder neck and since the prostatic urethra and anterior urethra were otherwise normal it was assumed that this blood vessel accounted for his haema-turia.

Over the next 3 years he had intermittent haematuria and at approximately yearly intervals he underwent further review cystoscopies, but no disease was found in the lower urinary tract. However, in time he developed obstructive lower urinary tract symptoms compounded by further hae-maturia and a repeat IVU was performed. This showed entirely normal upper urinary tracts but it was now evident that he had a sizeable postmicturition residue and a large prostatic projection on the cystogram phase of the IVU. The patient was informed that he had a rather vascular prostate which was obstructive and accounted for his nocturia and disturbed sleep pattern; therefore he agreed to undergo a transurethral resection of the prostate.

At the preliminary cystoscopy three benign-looking fronded papillomata, less than 1.5 cm in diameter, were found in the bladder. These were all resected, haemostasis secured and the fragments sucked out. Following this the resectoscope was exchanged (this is our normal practice but may in fact be unnecessary) to avoid the possibility of contaminating the prostate with transitional cells. Subsequently 40 g of prostate were resected and his postoperative recovery was uneventful. The bladder lesions were reported as Grade I transitional cell carcinoma and the prostatic tissue was entirely benign.

After finding transitional cell lesions in his bladder the patient was put on the review cystoscopy list at 3-monthly intervals and in the next 12 months underwent 3 review cystoscopies. During this time nothing more than a few mossy areas were found in his bladder all of which were cauterised.

Fifteen months following transurethral resection of the prostate he developed an attack of haematuria that persisted over a 3-week period. This became quite disconcerting to him and it was decided to carry out a further review cystoscopy, although it was only 6 weeks since the last one, when everything was found to be normal. At this repeat cystoscopy the bladder was entirely normal, as was the bladder neck, the prostatic cavity remained well healed and there was no evidence of transitional cell seedling of the prostatic cavity and the whole of the anterior urethra was normal. At cystoscopy both ureteric orifices looked normal but no urine was emerging from either side. The anaesthetist was invited to set up an intravenous infusion. The patient was given a litre of dextrose saline very quickly. A second litre was infused and he was given an injection of 20 mg of Lasix. Soon after, urine emerged from the left ureteric orifice and this seemed to be normal in colour but nothing emerged from the right. Then, at the height of inspiration, it was noted that the tip of a papilloma was protruding through the right ureteric orifice. With the small cupped biopsy forceps it was just possible to catch the tip of the protruding tissue for biopsy. A Chevassou catheter was then introduced into the ureteric orifice to perform an ascending ureterogram to determine the pathology present in the lower urinary tract. However, it was not possible to introduce the Chevassou catheter beyond 1 cm and the contrast ran back into the bladder. It was decided that it would be inappropriate to try and introduce the ureterorenoscope dilators or the instrument itself into the lower ureter.

An IVU was carried out several days later and this showed an entirely normal left renal tract. On the right side the nephrogram appeared late, there was a delay in the excretion, the calyces were slightly dilated and the upper ureter eventually filled down to approximately 3 to 4 cm above the vesico-ureteric junction. The lower 3 to 4 cm of the ureter did not fill at all and, at the cut off point, the contrast medium did not taper but was dome-shaped suggesting that the lower segment of the ureter was filled with a papillomatous lesion.

Questions

What treatment options are now open to the Surgeon?

Discussion

This man had already demonstrated a transitional cell instability and now he had a tumour at the lower end of the ureter. The biopsy of the tip of the tumour taken with the biopsy forceps had suggested that it was a Grade 1 transitional cell carcinoma. However, we were only dealing with the tip of the tumour and knew nothing about the base of it. Conventional therapy for transitional cell carcinoma at the lower end of the ureter is to carry out a nephroureterectomy. However, the histology from his previous bladder biopsies was always grade I and there was no reason to believe on the evidence of this that the tumour in the lower end of the ureter would be anything other than the same. The treatment options were discussed with the patient and he was very keen to save his right kidney because he was fearful of developing the same problem on the other side. In the circumstances it was decided to try and avoid a left nephroureterectomy but instead explore the lower ureter, resect it and subject it to frozen section histological examination. This would then be followed by a reimplantation of the ureter into an accessible part of the bladder with or without the assistance of a psoas hitch. The other treatment option might have been to carry out a Boari flap; however, this possibility was excluded as it would interfere with mucosa already known to be unstable. By contrast the psoas hitch remained a safer possibility if the segment of ureter that was left behind was too short to allow anastomosis to the bladder.

The patient was positioned lying flat and a grid iron incision made in the right loin. An extraperitoneal dissection was made to reveal the ureter, which was identified and cleaned. The lower 3 cm of it were thickened and dilated; however it was possible to palpate the upper end of the abnormality and also to identify visually the area of the ureter which was entirely normal. The normal part of the ureter was divided 1.5 cm above the abnormal part in order to remove the lower spindle together with a cuff of bladder. There was considerable periureteric fibrosis present and in order to get down to the base of the bladder it was necessary to sacrifice the vas as it crossed over the ureter at the base of the bladder. After this the bladder was opened and the right ureteric orifice was then identified and a plain catgut suture was placed across the ureteric orifice which was then tented up. Using a small blade the ureteric orifice was circumcised and the mucosa freed from the underlying tissues. The dissection was deepened on the bladder side into the bladder muscle and then, by a combination of dissection both inside and outside the bladder, the uretreic spindle was removed together with the ureteric orifice and a cuff of mucosa. This particular procedure is awkward to perform because it is not possible to have control of the lower ureteric spindle from outside and at the same time easily effect the dissection inside the bladder. The mucosa at the right ureteric orifice was susequently closed and the defect in the posterior bladder wall closed with interrupted Dexon sutures; the 3 stay sutures that had previously been placed (1 above and 1 on each side of the ureterovesical junction) were used to reinforce the latter closure.

The specimen was taken to a side table, opened longitudinally and inspected. It was found that there was a papilloma in the intramural part of the ureter and that it was on a stalk. The ureter at the level of the lesion showed evidence of periureteritis and some dilatation but the mucosa was entirely smooth. There was nothing to suggest that there was disease other than the papilloma in the ureter. The changes above the papilloma resulted from the obstruction which the papilloma caused at the lower end. The segment of ureter was sent for frozen section and the histology confirmed that we were dealing with a grade I transitional cell papilloma.

In the circumstances it was decided that it would be reasonable to try and reimplant the ureter into the bladder in an accessible place. All the instruments were changed and a fresh set brought to the table and the gloves and gowns of the surgeon were also changed. A psoas hitch procedure was carried out and this was not difficult because the posterior wall of the bladder on that side had already been dissected, to some extent, to allow the ureteric spindle to be removed. The bladder on the right side was hitched up as far as the pelvic brim and 3 deep sutures were placed in the wall of the bladder and sutured to the psoas muscle, there being no tension on the bladder. The ureter was dissected a short way proximally and the distal 0.5 cm resected again for histology purposes. A pledget was placed in the bladder which was tented in a proximal direction and using a size 15 blade the bladder wall was opened by cutting onto the pledget from the outside. Following this a stay suture was placed in the lower end of the ureter which was then threaded into the bladder to lie comfortably. It was placed in such a position that it might well allow access for future ureterorenoscopy. The side wall of the bladder was anastomosed to the outer wall of the ureter by placing 3 circumferential dexon sutures. There was not enough ureteric tissue to form a true nipple in the bladder by turning the mucosa back, therefore a simple mucosa to mucosa suture (after bivalving the ureter) was effected in the bladder using absorbable sutures. The neoureterocystostomy was carried out over a double-ended pigtail stent, the proximal end of which was placed in the renal pelvis with the distal end lying in the bladder. At the end of this anastomosis there was no tension on the ureter and it seemed to lie quite comfortably. A urethral catheter was passed into the bladder through the penis and the bladder was closed in 2 layers of dexon, the mucosa first and then all layers. The bladder was then irrigated using a Wardill syringe. There was no leakage at the cystostomy site but a little irrigating fluid seeped out at the back of the bladder where the ureter had been reimplanted. A single suture was required to close this defect. A tube drain was placed *in situ* in the pelvis to drain any seepage from the neoureterocystostomy and the area where the pelvic spindle had been resected. The patient who did not require a blood transfusion was given peroperative antibiotics. After 10 days the catheter was removed and he passed his urine well but, initially, with some frequency. The plan at that stage was to carry out an IVU at 3 months prior to a review cystoscopy.

The IVU was undertaken at 3 months after the operation. The left urinary tract remained normal. The right kidney functioned immediately and this was before any urine reached the bladder, so there was no possibility that the contrast seen in the kidney could have been siphoned back by the double ended pigtail stent. There were no obvious defects in the ureter and the ureter outlined surprisingly well despite having a pigtail stent in it. A review cystoscopy was performed and there was no evidence of recurrences in the bladder. The pigtail stent was removed without any difficulty and the area where the neoureterocystostomy was fashioned was noted for future reference.

This patient will continue to be followed up by regular IVUs and cystoscopies at 3-monthly intervals. The IVUs will be limited to show whether there is any recurrence in the ureter or not. It is also possible that in future we will be able to examine the ureter with the ureterorenoscope because the upper ureter has a straight run into the bladder. Although it will be slightly rigid there should not be any difficulty in inspecting it.

Should the patient develop a recurrence in the ureter it may be possible to deal with this endoscopically using the ureterorenoscope, but if he continues to develop repeated recurrences it may be necessary to offer him a nephroureterectomy. However, if the patient develops a recurrence in the renal pelvis it may be possible to control this by carrying out a percutaneous nephrostomy, then introducing the nephroscope directly into the renal pelvis and fulgurating the tumour using the same technique as that which has been described for the percutaneous removal of an upper ureteric calculus.

It is too early to say to what extent percutaneous and ureterorenoscopic therapy will keep tumours in the upper urinary tract under control and thus either obviate or delay the need for more oblative surgery such as nephroureterectomy.

Case 63

A 71-year-old male presented with rectal bleeding and some rectal dysfunction. There was no significant past medical or surgical history and, when questioned, the patient did not admit to any urinary symptoms. He lived alone and was not well nourished. Physical examination did not reveal any abdominal abnormality but he was found to have a large rectal carcinoma and a small benign prostate on rectal examination.

Question

How should this man be investigated?

Discussion

A full blood count revealed that he was slightly anaemic, his urea and electrolytes and biochemical profile were within normal limits and the liver function tests showed no significant abnormality. On chest X-ray changes consistent with chronic bronchitis and emphysema were seen, but there was no abnormality of the cardiac outline. The barium enema performed on an outpatient basis demonstrated a filling defect in the rectum and there was no obvious carcinoma higher up, although there was some evidence of diverticular disease. The rectal biopsy confirmed a diagnosis of a well differentiated adenocarcinoma which was lying quite low in the rectum on EUA; the rectum was mobile but the surrounding tumour mass was more extensive than had been assessed by simple rectal examination.

The plan of treatment was to perform, through a lower left paramedian and perineal incision, an abdomino-perineal resection of the recto-sigmoid area and to fashion a terminal colostomy in the left iliac fossa. This operation was successful, and initially there did not seem to be any major problems, but after 48 hours it became apparent that he was leaking fluid through his perineal wound. His urinary output (via a catheter) during the first 48 hours was low and it was now apparent that he had developed a urinary fistula which might have accounted for his excreting less urine than might have been expected. At this stage no urine was draining from the pelvic drain; however, urine did emerge from the pelvic drain on the third postoperative day.

Question

What investigations should be carried out to ascertain the site of the urinary fistula?

Discussion

The first consideration was that there might be a leak from the back of the bladder which could possibly have been devascularised or damaged during the dissection. Such an injury could have allowed a pool of urine to collect in the pelvis and subsequently burst out through the perineal wound. The simplest way of demonstrating whether this was a possibility or not was to instill some contrast medium through the urethral catheter into the bladder; this actually showed that the bladder outlined and filled very well and that there was no extravasation. Therefore it was probable that one or other of the ureters were damaged, more likely the left. An IVU was therefore performed and both kidneys were well shown. The whole of the right urinary tract was demonstrated indicating that there was no fistula on the right side. On the left side the kidney functioned well, the calyceal pattern was normal and the upper ureter was seen. The lower ureter was not seen but subsequently contrast medium was noted to be pooling in the lower abdomen in the area of the pelvic brim and also in the pelvis. This investigation indicated that the injury had occurred to the left ureter but little was revealed about its extent.

Consequently, a cystoscopy was carried out with a view to inserting a ureteric stent into the upper left renal tract in the hope that by splinting the ureter, healing might take place. Cystoscopy revealed a normal bladder and the small size of the prostate was confirmed endoscopically. A catheter was placed in the left ureteric orifice but this could only be inserted for about 2 cm after which it would not ascend any further. Contrast medium was injected into the left ureteric catheter but this was seen to extravasate into the pelvis.

By combining the pictures of the IVU with those of the attempted ascending ureterogram, it seemed that a segment of the pelvic spindle had been damaged at the original operation. It was also clear from the IVU that the left kidney was a much better kidney than the right one (which was somewhat shrunken in size and although it worked well, was scarred). By now the patient's blood urea and creatinine had started to rise and he continued to discharge urine through his perineum which gave rise to considerable nursing difficulties.

The histology of the removed recto-sigmoid bowel indicated a moderately well differentiated adenocarcinoma with extension of tumour through the wall of the bowel but the specimen did not contain any ureter, despite a specific request to check for this.

Question

What surgical procedures were open to the urologist?

Discussion

This man's prognosis was uncertain despite the facts but there was no evidence of metastatic disease within his abdomen. Nonetheless the urinary fistula (which was making nursing rather difficult and was having a depressive effect on the patient) had to be attended to. The prospect of placing a percutaneous nephrostomy tube in the kidney while occluding his upper ureter by means of a balloon catheter was discussed; but this would only have been a temporary manoeuvre and would not have provided a long-term solution. Since the patient had a colostomy on the left side, it was felt that he might not be able to cope with a nephrostomy tube also on the left side.

Consideration was given to embolising the left kidney at arteriography but since the left was the better of the two kidneys it was concluded that this was not the preferred treatment option. Also there was the distinct possibility that embolisation might not be entirely successful and that his fistula would continue to leak. In addition because the left kidney was the better of the two and because the patient was slightly uraemic with a raised creatinine level a left nephrectomy through a loin incision was not undertaken. Finally, it was decided that this man would have to undergo a further laparotomy with a view to closing his fistula, but beforehand we needed to be sure that he would be able to pass urine voluntarily. His urethral catheter was removed for a short time and he demonstrated reasonably well over a period of 24 hours that he could empty his bladder with control. A psoas hitch procedure to try and bridge the gap between a possible defect in the ureter and the bladder would probably not be feasible because of the amount of surgical reaction in his pelvis; for the same reason a Boari flap was not seriously considered to be a treatment choice. It was therefore decided that, if at all possible, a transuretero-ureterostomy might provide the option that would require the least dissection.

A preliminary cystoscopy was performed and a double-ended pigtail stent was inserted up the right ureter, the top end of which was placed in the renal pelvis and the bottom end in the bladder. The old laparotomy wound was then reopened and the urine that was lying in the anatomical pelvis was sucked out. It was clear that either a Boari flap or a psoas hitch would have been impractical because of an intensive reaction in the anatomical pelvis from the presence of urine over the previous 7 to 10 days. A dissection of the left lateral wall of the pelvis failed to reveal any ureter but eventually it was identified above the pelvic brim by the leak. The ureter distal to this down as far as the bladder was completely necrotic, and it was concluded that something had happened to its blood supply at the time of surgery.

This ureter was not too difficult to mobilise because of the colectomy that had been carried out and because the patient already had an end colostomy. The ureter was freed up despite much peri-ureteric reaction, and swung across underneath the mesocolon to the right side. The right ureter was dissected out and displaced medially. This was facilitated by the ureteric stent which had been positioned a short time previously. The end of the damaged ureter was freshened and a vertical incision made in the right ureter above the level of the pelvic brim. An end-to-side anastomosis using interrupted dexon was carried out over a distance of approximately 1 cm. This anastomosis was protected by a T-tube which was placed in the left ureter about 4 cm above the uretero-ureterostomy. A tube drain was placed down to the site and the wound closed using tension sutures. The patient was started on a course of antibiotics and a blood transfusion was also instituted.

Following this the patient made quite good headway, his perineal wound gradually began to granulate and the various infections which he developed were treated by antibiotics. Over a period of several weeks his general nutritional state improved and he was able to be discharged from hospital several months after his original presentation with rectal bleeding.

When they do happen, ureteric injuries occur at the time of oblative rectal surgery because part of the ureter is damaged at removal of the specimen. These are the most common injuries, although occasionally the ureter might be ligated circumferentially. Necrosis develops in a ureter several days after surgery resulting in a urinary fistula is the least common type of injury in either general or gynaecological surgery. This particular case demonstrates the dilemma that faces clinicians looking after a frail patient with malignant disease who has developed a fistula in a different system from the original pathology. The simplest mode of treatment might have been to remove the kidney on the affected side; however, this would have the disadvantage of removing healthy tissue.

Transuretero-ureterostomy requires little dissection, the disadvantage of this procedure is that, if the anastomosis does not hold, then there is the possibility that the good ureter might be permanently damaged by the surgical intervention; thus the patient might develop bilateral fistulae. However, using a double ended pigtail stent and a protective T-tube which is removed after approximately 10 days when the T-tubogram showed that there was no stenosis or leakage at the ureterostomy site, it turned out to be the operation of choice for this particular man.

Three months after surgery, his pigtail stent was removed through the bladder with the aid of a short-acting general anaesthetic. Ten days later an IVU showed that both kidneys were working well, despite the presence of some fullness of both ureters in the area of the uretero-ureterostomy anastomosis. The single stem of the right ureter below the anastomosis was unchanged when compared to the IVU taken after his abdomino-perineal resection.

Case 64

An 18-year-old woman presented with a history of recurrent urinary tract infections since childhood. These childhood infections had been treated with antibiotics over the years while she was attending a children's hospital. Physical examination revealed some tenderness over the bladder but no other abnormality. She was normotensive. The haematological and biochemical investigations were entirely normal but her urine contained some pus cells and *Escherichia coli* organisms. An IVU was essentially normal although there was a slight suggestion of fullness in the right urinary tract. The cystogram phase of the IVU was normal with the bladder filling, outlining and emptying completely. A cystoscopy was carried out sometime after the original MSU was reported as being infected and, at that time, a CSU showed some pus cells but no organisms. There was some inflammation of the mucosa consistent with a recent urinary tract infection. The capacity of the bladder at that cystoscopy was not recorded but an EUA revealed no abnormality.

Over the next 4 years she attended the outpatient clinic regularly and was frequently found to have a urinary infection, each of which was treated on its merits. However, on a few occasions her urine was found to be sterile. Some of the attacks of infection were complicated by haematuria and on other occasions she had pain in the left loin area with fever. She developed a sensitivity to the Penicillin group of drugs and could therefore no longer use these; additionally she developed leucodaenia following a course of Cotrimoxazole. Subsequently, she became pregnant and, interestingly, during pregnancy most of her urinary symptoms seemed to disappear. After delivery she developed another attack of pyelonephritis with cystitis again and she was referred for the first time for a urological opinion.

Physical examination revealed no abnormality and the biochemical and haematological tests were normal and her urine grew pus cells and *E. coli*. As she was fairly recently delivered of her child, it was decided to defer the IVU because the IVU findings might be misleading so soon after pregnancy. In the meantime some early morning urines were examined which excluded a diagnosis of tuberculosis.

At the appropriate time, approximately 6 months after the delivery of her child an IVU was performed; this was essentially normal so far as the upper urinary tracts were concerned. Neither did it show evidence of scarring in either kidney, and the bladder which seemed not as large in size as it was previously 4 years ago, filled, outlined and emptied reasonably well. Shortly after the IVU a cystoscopy was performed and strikingly, the capacity of the bladder was reduced. Despite marked mucosal injection a biopsy was not taken, although the bladder mucosa did not look typical of interstitial cystitis. A EUA of the pelvis revealed no abnormality. The patient continued having recurrent attacks of cystitis and required further courses of antibiotics and 2 years after the delivery of her child a further cystoscopy was carried out.

The bladder capacity at this time was only 225 ml despite repeated distensions. There was a linear tear on the dome of the bladder compatible with interstitial cystitis and a biopsy was taken. The histological examination revealed non-specific chronic inflammation and severe glandular metaplasia. Although interstitial cystitis was not a proven diagnosis, it was certainly suspected clinically.

The patient continued to have recurrent urinary infections and needed treatment. She was offered regular cystodistensions and 1 year later her bladder capacity had increased to 300 ml but by now there was very definite evidence of interstitial cystitis endoscopically. The bladder was thick-walled and spongy. Random biopsies of the mucosa of the bladder confirmed the diagnosis of interstitial cystitis.

Her treatment was aimed at eliminating infections as they arose and distending the bladder regularly. By now her symptoms were quite incapacitating as she was passing urine every 30–60 minutes round the clock. The introduction of oral steroids was entertained but as she was only 24 years old it was thought inadvisable to put her on this drug because she might have to remain on it for many years. By now she had been fitted with an IUCD for contraceptive purposes. Her bladder capacity did not increase with cystodistention and her functional capacity remained very small indeed. Her life was now being dominated by her bladder symptoms and she had become rather depressed.

Questions

What were the treatment options open to the surgeon?
Did surgery have anything to offer this woman?

Discussion

The surgical treatment options were either to carry out a urinary diversion or to perform an augmentation cystoplasty. She was emotionally unsuitable for a urinary diversion and, as an attractive woman with a young family, she did not want to wear an appliance on her abdominal wall. This option was only mentioned in conversation and never seriously considered for her. The remaining options included a colocystoplasty or a caecocystoplasty. Both these options were explained to her. She was apprehensive about having surgery but nonetheless enthusiastic that her symptoms might be relieved.

She was admitted to hospital for an augmentation cystoplasty and her bowel was prepared by giving her a 2-day course of Flagyl and Neomycin. An enema and high colonic washout was performed the day before surgery to clear the bowel of faecal content; the patient was then restricted to a fluid diet during that 24-hour period.

A midline suprapubic incision was fashioned; this revealed no abnormality within the abdominal cavity. The bladder seemed to be thick-walled and spongy and not very mobile. A routine appendicectomy was carried out and then the ileo-caecal area carefully examined. A Meckel's diverticulum was looked for and found not to be present. The terminal ileum was divided close to its junction with the caecum and a segment of bowel containing approximately 7.5 cm of the ileum and caecum were isolated on their own vascular pedicle, namely the ileocolic artery. The gastrointestinal tract was reconstituted by an ileocolonic anastomosis and this was done by closing the end of the ileum and joining the ileum to the colon, side-to-end in 2 layers. Through the ileum the ileocaecal segment was irrigated with normal saline until all the faecal content was removed. The ileocaecal segment was then rotated through 180° and brought down to lie in the pelvis.

Following this, the bladder was mobilised by dividing the peritoneum. Using 2 Babcock forceps the bladder was tented up on each side and a right-angled Haughton clamp placed across the tented up dome of the bladder. Using a knife, the bladder was sliced off above the clamp, and this tissue which contained the scarred dome was sent for histology. The open caecum was then approximated to the opened bladder and the caecum was sutured to the bladder circumferentially with 2 layers of dexon. The posterior layer was sutured first using the muscle of both organs and then the mucosa was sutured continuously. Finally the anterior anastomosis was performed at mucosal level and then the bladder muscle was anastomosed to the full thickness of the caecum. Through the still open blind end of the ileum, the caecocystoplasty was irrigated with normal saline to test the anastomosis which was found to be competent. (Previously a catheter had been placed in the bladder and was on continuous drainage.) The blind end of the ileum was then closed off with dexon. A tube drain was placed down to the pelvis and situated at the back of the bladder, was brought out in the left iliac fossa.

The patient's initial postoperative recovery was uneventful and it was intended to leave the catheter in for approximately 12 days. She was continued on antibiotics. On the tenth postoperative day she developed a small faecal fistula which discharged through the abdominal wound. As there was no constitutional upset it was decided to treat her conservatively. Oral intake was stopped and she was treated by parental nutrition for 5 days. The fistula healed and caused no further problems. The bladder dome which had been removed at the caecocystoplasty showed classical evidence of interstitial cystitis.

Over the next 12 months the patient coped well. Her bladder capacity increased and, although she did experience some bladder spasms, the pain was much less than it had been before surgery. However, she was still suffering from recurrent urinary tract infections. She was only getting up once per night to pass water compared with every 30–60 minutes previously, and she could hold on to her urine for several hours by day.

Much time was taken to explain to the patient and her general practitioner that it might take a very long time for the patient's urine to be rendered sterile. Once an augmentation cystoplasty was carried out it was quite likely that for some time to come organisms would be found in her urinary tract; this however did not mean that she was clinically infected.

Eighteen months following the augmentation cystoplasty her urinary tract was reinvestigated by means of an IVU and cystoscopy. The IVU showed that both upper urinary tract were unchanged and the bladder filled, outlined and emptied remarkably well at the end of micturition. At cysto-scopy, it was impossible to distinguish between the caecum and the bladder and the mucosa looked very healthy.

Here was a young woman who presented with urinary infections in childhood which persisted into early adulthood and gradually her bladder capacity became reduced. Initially the biopsy showed nothing more than chronic infection and inflammation in the bladder, but ultimately a diagnosis of interstitial cystitis was made both endoscopically and histologically. She was not offered steroids because she was so young but ultimately, because her bladder symptoms dominated her life, she was offered an augmentation cystoplasty. The augmentation ileo-caecocystoplasty was successful after an interval of time.

She was young to have undergone an augmentation cystoplasty and we were rather reluctant to offer her a urinary diversion. One of the problems with interstitial cystitis is that the bladder changes can develop in the bowel that has been superimposed on the bladder. When this happens the bladder and the bowel contract down again with a recurrence of the symptoms. Happily, some 6 years after her caecocystoplasty this has not happened and she is coping quite well despite the fact she still has occasional infections in her urine. She experiences some bladder spasms from time to time but these are reasonably well controlled with Urispas tablets.

At no stage was she offered steroid treatment because, once patients are put on steroids for interstitial cystitis, it is quite likely that they may become steroid-dependent. Classically, in interstitial cystitis the urine is sterile but this girl had a combination of infected urine almost all the time and a progressively shrinking bladder. Sterile pyuria is the normal bacteriological finding and so urinary tuberculosis has to be excluded.

Normal haematological values

Haemoglobin: Males   13.0–18.0 g/dl
           Females   11.5–16.5 g/dl

Red cell volume: Males	$4.5–6.5 \times 10^{12}/l$
Females	$3.8–5.8 \times 10^{12}/l$
Haematocrit: Males	0.40–0.54
Females	0.37–0.47
Mean cell volume:	80–97 fl
Mean cell haemoglobin:	27–32 pg
Mean cell haemoglobin concentration:	31–35 g/dl
Reticulocytes:	0.2–2.0%
Leucocytes:	$4.0–11.0 \times 10^{9}/l$
Platelets:	$150–400 \times 10^{9}/l$
Erythrocyte sedimentation rate: Males	0–5 mm/l
Females	0–7 mm/l
Neutrophils:	40–75%
Lymphocytes:	20–45%
Monocytes:	2–10%
Eosinophils:	1–6%
Basophils:	<1%

Normal biochemical ranges of values

Plasma/Serum

Albumin: ambulant	38–48 g/l
hospitalised	25–48 g/l
Bilirubin:	<22 µmol/l
Calcium:	2.3–2.7 mmol/l
Cholesterol:	3.6–7.2 mmol/l
Cortisol: am	140–700 nmol/l
pm	up to 140 nmol/l
Creatinine:	up to 110 µmol/l
Glucose: fasting	3.3–5.6 mmol/l
random	3.3–8.4 mmol/l
Immunoglobulins (lgG):	7.0–16.0 g/l
Iron:	7.0–29.0 µmol/l
Iron binding capacity (total):	45–70 µmol/l
Magnesium:	0.6–1.0 mmol/l
Phosphate:	0.7–1.4 mmol/l
Potassium:	3.5–5.0 mmol/l

Protein (total) ambulant:	60–80 g/l
Sodium:	132–144 mmol/l
Thyroxine (T_4):	50–135 nmol/l
Tri-iodothyronine (T_3):	1.1–3.2 nmol/l
TSH:	<8 m U/l
TBG:	14–30 ng/l
T_4: TGB ratio:	2.2–5.8
Triglycerides:	0.8–1.8 mmol/l
Urate:	0.17–0.48 mmol/l
Urea:	3.5–7.4 mmol/l

Enzymes

Acid phosphatase:	0.13–0.56 U/l
Alkaline phosphate:	70–330 U/l
Amylase:	70–300 U/l
ALT (GPT):	5–40 U/l
AST (GOT):	5–45 U/l
Gamma glutamyl transpeptidase	<65 U/l

Acid-Base State

pH	7.36–7.44
pCO_2	4.5–6.0 K Pa
pO_2	12.0–14.7 K Pa
Bicarbonate	24.0–30 mmol/l

Index